THE
GOSPEL
OF
JOY

PUBLISHED BY HEAD2HEART PTY LTD

ACN 088-184-810

ABN 42-058-710-952

Head2Heart Pty Ltd
C/- PACA
Suite 3, Level 8, North Tower
1-5 Railway St., Chatswood
NSW 2067 Australia
61 (0) 414 28 22 18
email: amanda@amandagore.com

Published by Head2Heart Pty Ltd
ABN 73 088 184 810

Distributed by Head2Heart Pty Ltd

For ordering information or special discounts for bulk purchases, please
contact Head2Heart Pty Ltd at amanda@amandagore.com.

Interior & cover design by Margery Cantor, Vermont USA.

ISBN 978-0-9818794-1-3

First edition
Printed in the Australia on acid-free paper

Contact Amanda Gore at amanda@amandagore.com
for any information regarding this book.

CONTENTS

NOTE: THE REAL AUTHORS OF THIS BOOK

Writing this book changed my life.

That may sound strange, since I am sure many people who write books have cathartic experiences or things that happen to them along the way that open their eyes, but it had never happened to me before.

I write this page to share some of my experiences with you—and to say a prayer that you too find the process of reading this book a blessing and that it helps you find your own path to joy, as writing it has done for me.

This whole book is dedicated to eliminating unhappiness, giving you more control over your moods and helping you soar through the clouds to God's sunshine above.

To give you a bit of background about me, 25 years ago, I was a physical therapist in Australia, working in sports medicine, ergonomics and occupational health. I had coauthored a book called *The Office Athlete* which prompted a meeting planner to invite me to a conference. Noted inspirational speaker Ron Tacchi was the emcee at the conference, and at the end of my session, he said, "You should be a speaker!" I answered, "What's a speaker?"

Ron then mentored me into the business, which in itself was a huge blessing. I have been speaking, consulting and writing since then about emotional intelligence, connection, the human spirit, communication and relationships. I came to the United States in 2000 and was blessed from the moment my feet hit the ground here!

The journey through writing this book has led me to a whole new dimension and understanding of life. I had the knowledge in my head of all the principles and ideas I elaborate on here prior to writing this book, but I did not truly know all of them; I did not have them embedded in my heart. I did not operate from those principles, although I tried to.

For example, I understood forgiveness as an intellectual concept that I knew was important, but I now *know* about it in my heart, comprehend it better and have actually experienced forgiveness—and being forgiven—although I am still working on both!

Instead of struggling with just writing about equanimity, I have had some blinding flashes of the obvious and can see many aspects of my life from a completely different level—and I am behaving differently, with more equanimity!

I did not create this book. I wrote it, of course, but really my mum, who passed away in 2006, and her "spiritual writing team" (which included Miss Steve, my English teacher for all my years in primary school, and Gracie) created it. I was just a scribe! Many people may find this hard to believe or imagine, but it's *my* belief system, and my experiences have shown me how alive my mum's spirit is!

Have you ever woken up with a crystal-clear thought or idea, seemingly out of nowhere? Well, one morning, almost a year after Mum passed, and after months of struggling with how to write this book, I woke up and I *knew* it was to be about joy; and I *knew* that the format it followed would be 12 weeks to joy; and I *knew* Mum and her team would help me; and I *knew* I had to meditate!

So I did, and each morning an idea would come to me and I would sit in silence with it and then go and write. It only took about two days for each chapter, as the words flowed easily out onto the pages. I could feel Mum, Gracie and Miss Steve and a host of others helping me in this process—it was an amazing experience!

I want to thank them for patiently teaching me such spectacular lessons which have made my life *much* more joyful.

And please note: Throughout this book, wherever I have written "God," if this is not appropriate for you, please replace it with the Divine,

Spirit, Universe, Source, Buddha, Allah, Love or whatever it is that *you* believe in.

I believe it's important that we all have the freedom to have faith in whatever we wish, even if it is just ourselves. (Although if your faith is *just* in yourself, you may wish to consider something a little bit bigger!)

THANKS MUM! I LOVE YOU.

DISCLAIMER

This publication is for information purposes only, and is designed as a general reference and catalyst to seeking further information about some aspects of self care. The authors and editors are not responsible for the results of any actions taken on the basis of any information in this publication, or for any error in or omission from this publication.

Neither the publisher nor the online publisher is engaged in giving medical or other advice or services. The publisher, online publisher, authors and editors, expressly disclaim all and any liability and responsibility to any person, whether a reader of this publication or not, in respect of anything, and of the consequences of anything done or omitted to be done by any such person in reliance, whether wholly or partially, upon the whole or any part of the content of this publication.

People should exercise their own independent skill or judgment or seek professional advice before relying on the information contained in this publication. No legal liability or responsibility for any injury, loss or damage incurred by the use of, or reliance on, or interpretation of, the information contained in this publication is accepted.

ACKNOWLEDGMENTS

There are a lot of people to thank for their contribution to, and influence on, this book. Just some of them are listed here. I am blessed to know them all and grateful for their amazing contributions to my life.

God

Mum – Lenore Lewis

Miss Steve

Ken Wright

Mary Forte

Kathy Warner & Bob Simmonds

Julianna Millar

Michael Grinder

Keith Harrell

Jennifer Griffin

The Poscentes

My Lord

Gracie

The Committee

Robert & Cheryl Sardello

Somer McCormick

The Simarts

Simon Gore, my brother

Dianne Hermans

Denise Rizzo

Brenda & Frank Bailey

SPECIAL ACKNOWLEDGMENTS

Robert and Cheryl Sardello from the School of Spiritual Psychology deserve a special mention for their contribution in developing my heart capacities, which are now clearly reflected in all I do. Through their writings and courses, many lives have changed or been transformed, including mine. Without their work, this book would have been very different. Thank you both with my whole heart. The website for the classes is www.spiritualschool.org.

Mary Forte's inspired guidance made the final book possible. Bless you and thank you Mary.

THE GOSPEL OF JOY

"Jubilation is the motto for future times.
In joy lies the greatest force."[1]

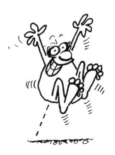

PROLOGUE

When I began writing this book, I wondered how on earth I would do it. Joy, when you really think about it, is not something we talk about much. Where would I start? What do *I* know about joy? How do you define it? How do you teach it? I had a million other questions.

My time frame was originally to write this book in February 2006, but life stepped in and my precious mother, Lenore Joan Lewis, a remarkable, courageous and beautiful woman, crossed the threshold that month.

It's now 36 months later, and my mother is with me still—helping me write this book! I have worked inwardly a great deal since she passed and I have come to realize that joy is both complex and simple at the same time.

In a nutshell, joy comes from a relationship with God and/or the Divine.

It is so simple to do the little things that accumulate and create a soul bursting with joy. It may not always be easy, but it *is* simple! Not much of what I write is new—we all know what needs to be done, but it's the *doing it* that is the challenge!

And that's the aim of this book—to give you small steps that you can take daily and weekly, each one of which shares with you a different aspect of joy; all of which lead you closer to living in joy.

Follow the ideas and exercises, and keep a journal. In 12 weeks, review your joy level. You might be amazed at how dramatically you have changed!

This book is a gift from my mother, both to you and to me.

Another gift in this process was the little farmhouse my husband and I found in Vermont. The peace, silence and beauty I have experienced here has been perfect for writing, and I know that my mother helped me to find this haven where I have been able to experience *my* journey to joy. Bless you and thank you Mama!

Love and giving thanks is the essence of this book—love and gratitude.

With joy, there is gratitude.
With gratitude, there is reverence.
With reverence, there is service.
With service, there is compassion.
With compassion, there is love.
In fact, with love we have everything to give!

INTRODUCTION

"This is the day the Lord has made and I will rejoice and be glad in it."

—Psalms 118:24

Joy is a gift from God for those who have a pure heart. When we have a pure heart—one that wants only good for everybody, sees God in everyone and everything, and seeks opportunities to bring God into the world—we can feel joy. Fear stops us from feeling joy.

Joy is like a hologram. No matter how many pieces the hologram image breaks into, the whole is always within the piece. We are born with the capacity for joy—we are a piece of the hologram, yet whole. Our life journey is to realize that the whole is available to us—it's not necessarily in us now, but we can stretch out our hand and receive joy. We are given the whole when we receive this joy and then give through serving others. We are to strive to manifest the whole. We can develop the sacred capacity to see and experience the whole in all the other pieces called humans! That is the condition where true joy lives.

HOW TO USE THIS BOOK

1. You can read it all the way through and then simply work with the chapters that resonate with you. Or you can read it all the way through and contemplate what you want. Or you can skim through it and just

pick out areas that you would like to work on when and where you want to work on them!

2. You can open it at random. Focus on what you find on that page. It is fascinating how often *that* page can have a particular meaning for you at that moment.

3. You can just dive in and make this a planned journey to joy. Do this by yourself or with your family. Working through the book and doing the exercises alone or together can lead to amazing insights because we are actually *practicing* something, even if we don't think the practice will help.

Each week, there will be a new concept or feeling to work with. Select the day of the week when you would like to start each week's journey. I have chosen Sunday as the start day, but you can choose whatever works for you. On that day, begin with seven minutes of contemplation of the idea presented. (Why seven minutes? It doesn't have to be, of course, but that amount of time does provide structure.)

For example, the first week's focus is on gratitude.

Read the segment on gratitude. Then, on your chosen day, sit quietly somewhere and read the accompanying questions, reflect on gratitude and what it means to you, and think about what role it plays in your life.

A NOTE ON THINKING & CHOICES

Thinking happens in your heart. Put your attention in your heart. Ask the questions *from* your heart. Then listen *to* your heart.

It may help to consider that we seem to do all our thinking and self-talk in our heads, but our hearts really control our thinking and behavior.

Do you remember the old cartoons that had a character with a little devil sitting on one shoulder and an angel on the other? This is how I imagine thinking with our heart operates. We have an imaginary "strategy box" sitting above our left shoulder and a "conscience box" above our right, and both of them are connected to our heart. Each is trying to influence our actions.

The heart "thinks" by receiving input from each box, and then it makes a choice as to what our right action or behavior will be. Our hearts need to choose to follow divine inspiration, which comes through the "conscience box." It is wise to consciously filter all our decisions through the "conscience box" because the heart seeks information on ways to behave from the "strategy box." If a faulty program is installed in the "strategy box," our hearts continue to make unwise decisions and our behaviors remain the same. We need to become conscious of these faulty programs and "self talk" and filter every choice we make through the "conscience box."

Among many other factors, our choices can be influenced by our environment—by what we saw our parents do or by our genes. We must learn to make the right choices, the God-inspired choices. If we ask for help and listen to God, He will always guide us wisely. It is through our hearts and bodies that we feel and experience everything. When our hearts make wise choices, we feel calm and peaceful. A churning stomach is often a sign of a poor choice of strategy!

We rarely understand the significance of our heart—until it stops working. What happens then? We die! Remember, we can be brain-dead and still alive, but since the physical body needs oxygen, once our heart stops, we cannot survive. The spiritual heart is the portal for God's love, pumping the life forces of divine love through our beings. The spiritual body needs to love and to have love.

One technique that I'm going to refer to throughout this book has to do with learning how to "drop" to your heart to receive guidance. I have done this unconsciously in the past, but I learned so much more about the technique and its impact from Robert and Cheryl Sardello. I'll talk more about this later, but at its simplest, this is how it works:

To "think" with your heart and hear the heart's guidance, find a quiet spot (if needed) and become aware of the area around your heart. Focus on that area and see if you can "drop" your attention down to that part. Then imagine you are breathing through your heart, that the breath flows in and out through your heart.

As you continue to do that for a few minutes, a sense of peace and calm may flow through you. You may feel safe and secure, and after a time, there will be a sense of "knowing" what you need to do in a particular situation. You may also find that words appear to you—they just emerge into your consciousness. Or perhaps an image will float through that gives you an answer you needed or some insight that solves a difficulty for you. You may even feel a sense of compassion that helps you understand why another person is acting the way they are, and that will help you resolve a problem. A brilliant idea may even "pop" into your thinking! That's the way the heart works—it is subtle, kind and usually very wise.

Take a little time now to practice this exercise. You only need about five minutes at a time—or even less if you don't have five minutes. Once you are used to this, it takes only a few seconds to have heart consciousness and access to that wisdom and love.

Another way you may be able to enter into your heart is by imagining a chute—like a laundry chute—going from the top of your head down through your body to the center of your heart. Imagine a miniature you sliding down the chute and landing gently in the interior space of your heart. Just put yourself in there and stay and rest a while in the silence and peace.

Keeping a journal is a great idea during your 12-week journey to joy, as you will be amazed at the heart insights that emerge! Make notes on what you have learned and how it affected you at the end of the week or each day. And just as importantly, note how your changes in behavior or thinking affected others around you.

When you have finished working through this book, what you have written will create your own journey to joy!

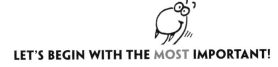

LET'S BEGIN WITH THE MOST IMPORTANT!

A WEEK OF **GRATITUDE**

"What you want is so near, so near!
It requires only the little shift,
The simple turn, from self to higher,
The letting go of time, worries, doubts.
Let the spirit of gratitude carry you."[1]

—Claire Blatchford

Actually, it would be better if I suggested living a *life* of gratitude, not just a week. But a week is a great place to start. It is difficult in our fast-paced society to focus for one day on gratitude, let alone a week! For some, this will represent a new way of being in the world and can be transformational—it's amazing what sincere gratitude can do.

YOUR SEVEN MINUTES

Take your seven minutes now to reflect on how gratitude plays a part in your life.

What does gratitude mean to you?

Do you feel grateful a lot of the time?

Are you grateful for many things?

To whom and for what are you grateful?

What types of things make you feel grateful?

Did your parents' behavior model gratitude?

Did your siblings or another adult model gratitude as a way of living?

What have you been really thankful for in your life?

It may be difficult to answer these questions truthfully, but take the time and really think (consciously, with your heart) about the things in your life that bring about in you a feeling of gratitude. If you don't think about gratitude much at all, it's okay! The world we live in does not leave much time or space to enter into gratitude.

Now is the time to create an opening in your life to feel gratitude and allow it to flow freely. This will have an amazing effect on how you view, and exist in, the world. It will also help others as they become aware of gratitude just by seeing your transformation. This is a VERY important week for all of us.

AMANDA'S TAKE ON GRATITUDE

"To speak gratitude is courteous and pleasant, to enact gratitude is generous and noble, but to live gratitude is to touch Heaven."[2]

—J. A. Gaertner

A GRATITUDE JOURNAL

My most poignant story of gratitude is about my mother. She was living in Australia when I had moved to the United States. She was lonely, unhappy, unwell and in pain, and I felt so bad about not being there to help and support her. She never complained about her problems or about missing me, but I know it was a huge struggle for her. It still causes me pain to think of how I was not there for her in person.

One day, when she was particularly down, I said, "Mama, why don't you make a list of things for which you are grateful every day? Spend ten minutes reflecting on that list every night before you sleep, and do it during the day if you feel lousy." We spoke of this idea for a few nights and then I forgot about it. It did seem to help her though, as she seemed happier for a while after that.

I was going through her belongings after she died and found a little spiral-bound notebook that she had used as her gratitude book. I still have not been able to read it all. Just thinking about it brings me to tears because she tried so hard! The effort it took her to write is obvious; her handwriting looks as if her hand was trembling, and the words are hard to read. And she really did keep up her notebook for a long time. She never made a big deal of it—that was her way. She would try everything in an effort to grow, to be free of pain, and to be joyful and more active. So if *she* can write a gratitude journal with *all* the problems she had, so can we!

For me, gratitude is something with which my mother blessed me. I have always been grateful for anything anyone does for me, or for benefits that come along—maybe because I don't expect such things, and so they are always a gift.

When I was a little girl, we did not have much money. I knew we were in difficult circumstances. My parents were divorced when it was not a common practice and my father was an alcoholic, but I always seemed to have what I wanted or needed. My mother would wake up every morning at 4 a.m. to go to work so she could then come home, take us to school, and be at home when we came home. She made great sacrifices for us and I have always been grateful to her. I think knowing that, and knowing how hard she worked to give her children great schooling and everything they needed, has made me appreciate everything that comes to me—from anyone.

Some people have never experienced gratitude or had it modeled for them by their parents or other adults when they were growing up. Those people may find this work on discovering, developing and embracing their gratitude challenging, but it's worth the effort. By doing this, a whole new dimension is added to life.

If we think only of ourselves and expect the world or others to provide what we need, if we fail to see the world through others' eyes as well as our own, life becomes a battleground over what we want and what we have.

Gratitude gently leads us to an awareness of others and their needs, helps our hearts and souls expand, and ultimately fulfills us more than we could have imagined. It's not "things" that feed our deepest needs—it's love and gratitude.

Gratitude is the opposite of selfishness. It is a view away from the self. It is seeing and appreciating anything that is given to you, especially what *others* have given you, done for you or sacrificed for you. If nothing else, knowing that we are blessed with God's grace every moment, even though we may not deserve it, is enough to keep me eternally grateful.

COUNT YOUR BLESSINGS

Blessings come *as a result* of using the spiritual gifts we have been given to overcome challenges, hardships or "burdens." Receiving spiritual gifts, and then *doing something* with those gifts, allows us to deal with difficulties. Bad things happen, but God takes everything and makes it work out for the good. If we receive Divine inspiration and exercise our gifts, God blesses us so we can then go and bless others.

Even when I have to struggle to find something for which to be grateful, I do it. When something bad happens or I encounter a challenge or difficulty in life, I try to conclude my thinking with, "Well, I *am* grateful for . . ."

For example, I had a *very* difficult time once with the customer service hulk (I can't say "department"—it's just too big) of a particular software company. After about six hours of being shafted from one country and service person to another—none of whom knew anything outside of their narrow area of expertise—I still had a nonworking computer, and I was ready to kill someone! I hung up the phone and screamed.

After several hours, I was finally able to feel immense gratitude that I also owned another brand of computer! I know, I should have recognized my gratitude immediately, but it was only when I calmed down that I was able to feel thankful.

I felt thankful because I learned a lot through that experience. I learned patience, perseverance, tolerance and the capacity to separate the person to whom I was speaking from the difficulty I was facing. I also learned to realize that *what I was thinking* and how I was behaving were increasing my frustration more than anything! In any painful situation, we are given wonderful opportunities to find out more about ourselves and to practice being kind and tolerant, if not loving.

Of course, each time I have been through one of these frustrating experiences, I ultimately understand that it's all about me and how I respond to the experience—in other words, how I manage myself, and the choices I make. This isn't such an easy lesson, but whenever we point a finger at another, there are three fingers pointing back at us! No matter how much I wanted to, I could not blame anyone else for my reaction.

Sometimes we have to look really hard to find something for which to be thankful, but it's worth the effort. It's better for your nervous system, for those around you, for relationships and generally for life! Being grateful is a direct path to joy. Things we see as negative almost always lead to some type of blessing. Before you judge something that happens to you as horrendous—even if it truly is—try to imagine how this might be an opportunity for God to bless you.

We never really know, after all.

For example, I have a friend named "Lady Dianne," about whom you will read more later. She was scheduled to have surgery to remove a tumor, but the night before the proposed surgery, the endocrinologist said she could not proceed since she might have Cushing's disease, a condition where the adrenal glands do not work. Had the surgery proceeded as scheduled, her body may have failed to recover even if the surgery was successful.

Despite the pretty nasty symptoms she was living with daily, Dianne's surgery was put off for two weeks. But how did the amazing Dianne look at this? As a blessing! She said she was thrilled, as it gave her two more weeks to strengthen her adrenals before the surgery and to allow alternative strategies to work. She even laughed as she now had "an official reason to rest." But wait, there's more!

Dianne was in the hospital anticipating her surgery when the neurosurgeon told her to go home. Since it was already 8 p.m., this was unusual, as normally the patient would stay overnight and go home the next day. Instead, she went home and slept beside her six-year-old daughter, with whom she is very close. During the night, her daughter had an attack of croup that was so bad she went into respiratory distress. The child could have died had Dianne not been there.

What may have looked like an almighty problem—Cushing's disease—instead held within its hands the gift of Dianne's daughter's life.

My personal experience (and Dianne's) is that God makes everything work out for the good—especially for those who love Him. If your heart is on God, as Dianne's was and is, He will guide you through.

LOOK FOR THE GIFT

> "Only an open heart understands that everyone who enters our life is a guest bearing a gift. Sometimes we must seek out the gift."[3]
>
> —Susan L. Taylor

A book that changed my life is *Illusions* by Richard Bach. (The full title is *Illusions: The Adventure of a Reluctant Messiah*; published by Random House.) There is a line in the book that says something like, "Every problem bears a gift in its hand for you—look for that gift." And ever since I read that, I have!

Our past or current life partners, siblings, parents and friends—all of them have been "sent" to us with precious gifts, including the gift of spiritual growth. These gifts come whether we consciously want them or not!

Bless each of your relationships and be grateful to and for them, as they teach us character-building life lessons that no one else is willing to. (And remember, it may not always be the most pleasant experience for them, either!) We, in turn, also give them valuable gifts with the learning opportunities we offer them.

When we are with people with whom we interact easily and it's always fun, we may not be offered as many opportunities for growth. Do people who always agree with us challenge us to learn? Probably, but I suspect our greatest growth comes from the periods of trials and difficulties—where we *have* to stretch ourselves and be uncomfortable for a time in order to learn and change.

In every difficult relationship or experience you have, look for the gift. Find something in what is happening for which to be thankful— even if it is only that you are still breathing!

When I was 45, I lost all the money I had worked very hard to earn through a bad business venture. And although that whole ordeal took five years, involved long, nasty court cases, was extremely stressful, and caused me to move to another country and be away from my family, I was blessed by it.

I would never have had the opportunity to work in the United States if it had not happened. And this journey in the U.S. has been one of great growth for me. True, some of that growth has been very hard, but all of it is useful and has led to experiences I would never have had if I had not lost all the money.

If you feel everything about your life is miserable, be grateful you have the capacity to change things, even if it is only your thinking that you change. In fact, that is the *first* place to start!

How you choose to perceive things or the expectations you hold will determine what you see and how you feel. You can think your life is miserable, or you can realize you have free will and then you can *choose* to make whatever changes you want. Be grateful you have the gift of free will, but remember, it comes with responsibility.

If your life is other than you would like, and all the people around you are horrible, remember that *you* played a role in creating this situation, and *you* have an opportunity to make changes that will improve it, remove it or change it. You have the power to pray, to change your thoughts and thinking process, and, often with the help of others, to change your circumstances, *if you so choose.*

We need to make the choice to seek a life change, not knowing what will emerge or unfold, but trusting and praying for God to inspire us with what to do and give us opportunities to do it. And then *we* need to do it. Listen carefully for that intuition—"the inner-tuition"—from your heart. Our pure hearts inspire us with the *right* things to do—it's up to us to use our free will to do them or not.

For example, no one wants to die telling others, "Don't do what I did." When you look in the mirror at the end of your life, you want to see a life, and a heart, full of love. You want to know you loved as often and as well as you could—not fearing hurt, rejection or whether people loved you back. Although this may not be easy, we are all born with the abilities and gifts to do God's will, as well as with the capacity for free will—which is where our most important choices are made.

Changing your heart changes your thinking. No one needs to know you are changing your thoughts about your life, yet it is an extremely powerful thing to do, particularly if you are in circumstances that stop you from making actual physical changes.

There is *always* something you can do. There are places and people to go to and ask for help; mental strategies you can create; exercises you can do; health practitioners to see if you have imbalances. Just *do something* to change your circumstances. Ask God for guidance, and ask others for guidance and help. In the meantime, change what you are saying to yourself about the situation you are in—that can change everything else.

Reflect on what is currently happening to you, and look for the lessons, be thankful for them and learn from them. Choose to believe that in time, you will receive blessings from what you are going through.

You may have to learn courage or the capacity to stand up for yourself; or to learn that you actually *can* change your thinking and it *does* change your life. Or perhaps you are meant to be learning patience, kindness or compassion, or that you are not responsible for other adults' actions, or one of the many other concepts discussed in this book.

Only *you* will know what gifts you need that have come packaged in seemingly tough lessons!

LOSING SOMEONE YOU LOVE

If something really tough happens—like someone you love dies—grieve and mourn, but as quickly as you can, focus on how grateful you are to them.

After Mama died, I found that when I grieved, it was really for *me* and I wasn't able to feel her close to me. But when I focused on sending her love and gratitude, I could feel her presence and had a sense of peace. I am sure she did not want to see me suffering, missing her and feeling pain. I am sure your loved ones don't want to see you in pain either. They are probably going through a challenging enough time working out where they are and what they need to be doing without having to worry about us grieving over them!

When I focused on sending Mama my love and gratitude for all she had done for me, it *seemed like* I was giving her more of a gift, although in reality, it was helping me to stop wallowing over *my* loss! Of course I still mourn and grieve, especially as I write this book on the second anniversary of her death, but I only let those feelings flow for a short time. I consciously focus on sending Mama my love and gratitude, and soon I am feeling better and I can feel her again. I hope it helps her as well.

Through the pain of your loss, be grateful that you had time with your loved one in their earthly form. And they may not have left anyway! My belief is that our loved one's spirit may no longer be encased in a human body, but his or her spirit is still with us in a different state. Be grateful for their life and the extraordinary gifts you received. Focus on what you had rather than what you have lost or the regrets you have. Then send the person love and thanks for everything they did for you. Honor the ones who have passed with love, gratitude and joy.

If you are still having trouble finding something for which to be grateful, you may want to skip ahead and read the week on forgiveness. I, like many others, had one fabulous parent and one absent, rather difficult one. Both of them taught me invaluable lessons—it just took longer to understand the ones from my father. The primary lesson I took from him was true forgiveness; it took me a long time to learn it, but when I did, it had a huge impact.

BE A GOOD FINDER

> "If you concentrate on finding whatever is good in every situation, you will discover that your life will suddenly be filled with gratitude, a feeling that nurtures the soul."[4]
>
> —Rabbi Harold Kushner

Our pastor, Mark Craig, is an amazing storyteller. He once told of a research project where the scientists hoped to find the secret of success by studying a thousand "successful" people. The scientists were stunned by their conclusion: the common denominator with all these people was not education or socioeconomic status or parental wealth, but that they were all "good finders." The researchers invented this term to describe how these very successful people looked at the world.

In every person and every situation, these successful people found the good and *actively looked for* the good.

Interestingly, as I was writing this, I made a typo and said they looked for *God*. I don't think that was a mistake! Maybe the secret is to be a good finder *and* a God finder. When we are constantly finding God or good, it's easy to be grateful. *Everything* is a blessing when we see the world through gratitude.

What is your "nature"? Are you "naturally" optimistic—do you have a "happy" gene? Or do you think of yourself as skeptical? Pessimistic? Do you let things weigh you down? Do you always see the bad potential consequences of everything? Are you fearful most of the time?

Many people who have had difficult challenges in life have *learned* to be pessimistic (based on their fear). But we are not born pessimistic! Babies don't pop out and say, "Life is horrible!"

We are *all born with the capacity for joy*. Our job, as adults, is to find that kernel of joy already present and nurture it. Try to find and nurture your joy day by day this week. Once you start, it can become a lot easier. If it's a struggle to find your joy, pray and ask God to help you.

When we told people about our move to Vermont, many of them made negative comments: "You'll freeze; it will be so cold; you think it's good now, but wait til the snow hits" or "Wait til mud season!" Very few said, "What an exciting adventure!" or "How beautiful and peaceful it will be!"

None of us has to listen to pessimistic people. Who wants to hear that the glass is half empty when it *really is half full!* You can change how you view things—if you really want to.

Here is your challenge: With every single thing that happens this week, find something—no matter how small—that is good about it. Find something good about every single person you meet. Know that you can learn optimism. (There is a wonderful book by Martin Seligman called *Learned Optimism: How to Change Your Mind and Your Life,* so if you need help, that's a starting point.)

The best way to tackle finding something good about people and situations is to first catch yourself when you are being negative. Become aware of how much you fall into that trap, and start working on recognizing those negative thoughts *before* they have taken over. Replace them with "good finder" thoughts!

Find as many good things as you can about your life. Find something good about your home, your car or your financial situation. Find something good about every single person in your immediate family and every colleague at work. Focus on only the good for this whole week. (Actually, if you did it for a month or a year, that would be even better!) Consider putting a note on your computer that says, "I AM A GOOD FINDER," in case you need reminding!

REFRAME

Have you ever taken a picture to the framing store to select a mount and frame? I am always amazed at how a different frame can transform a painting, making it vibrant and alive or sucking the life out of it!

We can do the same thing for ourselves with words. If we hear someone say something negative, we can immediately reframe what that person said in our own thoughts, which changes the impact their words have. (It may help to think of what that person was *intending* to say—the real message behind the words.)

For example, what if someone says, "We'll never have this done in time." Instead of taking their fear or anxiety on board and feeling your stress and pressure mount, say, "This is a great chance to see how much we can achieve under pressure. What an opportunity!"

If you utter or think the words, "We'll never have this done in time," your body-mind immediately goes into stress mode. Stress chemicals pour out and pump through you, making you less efficient and affecting your thinking and capacity to be clear and creative. This causes you to lose sight of the bigger picture.

On the other hand, if you choose to reframe the situation through your words, you have a completely different mind-set and "body set"— you have different chemicals racing around your body, ones that will help you focus and do the job. It's simple and effective!

Consider this: A friend of mine had to go to the dentist for a crown. She could not have anesthesia because she is allergic to it. Unthinkingly, I said, "Oh, that must have been terrible!" She replied, "It's not nearly as bad as the effect of the anesthesia!"

There are many ways we can reframe the words we use to make them beneficial for us and to help us feel gratitude. Catch your own and others' phrases that pull you down, and replace them with a reframed version.

As I mentioned earlier, my great friend in Australia, Dianne (or as she laughingly calls herself "Lady Dianne"), was recently diagnosed with a pituitary tumor. (That's a pretty serious brain tumor.) She initially lost some sight in her left eye, and had terrible headaches and diminished sensation on the left side of her body. Instead of succumbing to terror and fear as most people would, she has felt those emotions but has also used her will to laugh her way through her challenges.

As I wrote earlier, she said that now she had an "official reason" to take a rest. As a mother of two small children, and as someone who is running one business and developing another with her husband, and who is *also* studying for her master's, she has a bazillion reasons to rest!

In my opinion, shared by many others, she is an angel and a queen of reframing. She has found good in a terrible situation and focused on that with laughter. Her chance of recovery is much greater than that of someone who succumbs to fear and pain.

Take whatever happens to you and go through the negative to the gift within it—that's what reframing is all about.

WEAR "GRATITUDE GLASSES"

It is impossible to have a heart full of misery and a heart full of gratitude at the same time.

Do you recall the old saying about people who see through rose-colored glasses, meaning everything they see looks rosy, pink, happy and good? Well, I believe there are people who walk around wearing black glasses! It doesn't matter what is really there—they see black in everything because of how they look at it.

I would like to introduce the concept of "gratitude glasses." Put them on every morning and do not take them off til you go to sleep that night.

What color glasses are you wearing: Black? Rose? Bored? Angry? Frustrated? Lonely? Miserable? Disappointed? Resentful? Poor me? Cynical? Resigned? Compassionate? Or gratitude?

I am so glad I have chosen to see the world and people through mostly rosy gratitude glasses—although it is something I work on daily. Good finders do not wear black glasses!

Go out today and buy yourself a pair of children's plastic sunglasses—preferably heart shaped. Knock the dark lenses out of them and wear them!

Okay, if you are not brave enough to *actually* wear them, buy them and put them on your desk. Have a second set for the car and a third for home and maybe a fourth for beside the bed. These can be your gratitude glasses. (If you can't find any, we have them on my website, www.amandagore.com. I use them to see through the "eyes of my heart.")

If you are feeling miserable, lonely, sad or depressed, consciously shift your attention to finding things for which to be grateful or appreciative. Put on your gratitude glasses! You will be amazed at how quickly you feel better. If nothing else, people will smile at you, and if you explain why you are wearing the glasses, they will probably ask for a pair!

This is another powerful tip: If you can't sleep, or have trouble sleeping, do this just before you go to bed. Instead of watching some soul-disturbing television program, lie quietly in bed and reflect on your day. Find three things for which you are grateful and focus on them until you fall asleep.

Put your gratitude glasses on if necessary—or maybe you need to put them on for your partner. Or you can both put them on! It may help to write down the things for which you are grateful in a gratitude journal, which you can keep beside your bed and make part of your nightly ritual. That's the way my mama did it.

When you wake up, immediately find something for which to be grateful. It will transform the nature of your day.

EXAMPLES OF SEEING YOUR WORLD
THROUGH GRATITUDE GLASSES (GG)

♥ GG help you see traffic delays as happen-ing for a good reason and possibly keeping you safe.

♥ GG wearers make the house they live in a home no matter how "bad" it is.

♥ GG wearers are grateful they have a family—even a dysfunctional one!

♥ GG folks see themselves as rich no matter how much money they have.

♥ GG alter the way you view what happened to you as a child. Filter what your parents did to you and for you through GG— you may be stronger, more resilient, more compassionate, and more loving as a result of your experiences.

♥ Seeing our food through GG reminds us to bless every meal and to be thankful for it and for those who prepared it for us.

♥ GG wearers are always reviewing their blessings and giving thanks for them.

THE ULTIMATE HEALING TOOL

"God gave you a gift of 86,400 seconds today. Have you used one of them to say thank you?"

—William A. Ward

The ultimate healing tool, along with forgiveness, is gratitude to God. If you can find it in your heart to be grateful to God for all you are and are not, all you have or don't have, and all that happens to you, you will know joy.

There *is* a reason for everything. We may never know why something happened, but we know that God can always turn situations around for those with a pure heart who have faith in Him. "Stuff" happens and it can be a trigger for us to learn, grow, be and do more with the help of God. *How we respond* to situations is most important.

If you don't agree with this, think of two people in similar circumstances, or who are afflicted with the same disease. Why does one survive and one not? Or of two people in a concentration camp? Why did Dr. Viktor Frankl, author of *Man's Search for Meaning,* live through his incarceration in a Nazi concentration camp while others did not? Why do some people suffer abuse in childhood and move on to lead fulfilling and successful lives with good relationships, while others live the rest of their lives bitter and angry?

I am not judging any of this—just pointing out that we always have free will and the ability to choose how we react, feel, think and live. There is *always* a choice. It may be very painful, it may take great personal courage, resilience, counseling, persistence and love, but no matter how we perceive it, we always have a choice—even if it's only a choice over how we think, feel and behave.

It may help you to read stories or view DVDs from people who have lived through horrendous or difficult circumstances to see how they have been able to deal with their past and how they learned to acknowledge and cope with their feelings to either emerge whole and healed, or to move on and enjoy their lives without complete resolution.

To paraphrase the bumper sticker on a friend's car: "Life is the teacher; gratitude, forgiveness and love are the lessons." Or maybe it's even simpler: "Life is the teacher, God is the lesson!"

Make it a ritual to come up with at least five things for which to be grateful each day, and hopefully many, many more. Remember, you are a good finder, a God finder! That makes it easy to find things for which to be grateful.

DAILY SCHEDULE

SUNDAY: GRATITUDE TO GOD

"I thank God for my handicaps for, through them, I have found myself, my work and my God."[5]

—Helen Keller

Isn't it amazing how a power outage in winter can make us *so* grateful for the power that surges through our houses every day? That invisible power gives us food, warmth, light and a comfortable life.

Hmmm ... what else is like that, I wonder?

Of course—it's God! (Or the Divine, Spirit, Source, whatever works for you.) God surges invisibly through us and around us all the time, healing us, "powering" us up, blessing us, pouring His grace into us, filling us with light, warming us, holding us, inspiring us, supporting us, guiding us, nourishing us and loving us.

He (I am using the term "He," but feel free to use whatever reference works for you here—we all have free will!) might use guardian angels or other people as angels to do some of His nurturing work. He can turn situations into something good for us, or send help or teachers in all sorts of shapes and sizes, or whatever is needed for us at that time.

Today, find reasons to be grateful to God and your angels. This should be an easy one!

Think what fun it would be if you identified all the angels in your life who are helping you right now. Look for them. Acknowledge your guardian angels and other spiritual and human beings who are working for you, with you and helping you.

We spend a lot of time in prayer *asking* God and our angels for help—for them to fix things and take this or that away or *do* something for us. What if we spent some time today and every day just listening, and asking what we can do for them? And in simply being grateful for everything they do for us?

Perhaps we can be of service to God and our angels in some way by being kind to another person or healing a broken relationship or forgiving someone—who knows what it could be. But I bet it would be interesting if you just sat and quietly listened for seven minutes. Or longer!

And for those of you who don't believe in prayer, what is the first thing most of us do if there is a life-threatening crisis? If we are suddenly diagnosed with a disease or worse, our child is? We pray! It's amazing how prayer comes into a person's life in those situations. And helps. Why wait for a disaster—begin now!

In my opinion, seeing God's influence on, and in, your life is essential for joy. Without this connection, there is no joy. When we feel truly grateful and connected to God, we are in a state of joy.

Remember, babies are born with a capacity for joy, but some action must happen for the joy to emerge. As soon as babies can actually "do" things, they become joyful. When we permit babies and toddlers the freedom to explore and accomplish new movements or tasks, we can see the joy in their faces. As we age and learn to use our spiritual gifts, joy flows into us and shows in our faces as well. We can rejoice with others who are in a state of joy—it can be contagious.

This day, focus on God and gratitude for everything He and His helpers do in your life. This should be an easy day with a lot of writing in your journal.

MONDAY: **WORKPLACE GRATITUDE**

"We often take for granted the very things that most deserve our gratitude."

—Cynthia Ozick

What things are you thankful for in your place of work? Go to work today with the specific intention of finding all the things you could be thankful for—and then *be* thankful for them! Your boss, your friends, your colleagues, the intellectual stimulation, the chance to learn, grow and develop, the relationships, the people you meet, the challenge of your work—there are many, many things for which you may choose to be thankful.

If you don't like your work or the people with whom you work, be grateful anyway. Actively *look for* things for which to be grateful—even if it is simply, "I am grateful that I am not out in the cold or hot or rainy weather. I am grateful I have a roof over my head. I am grateful I am paid for this." (Remember that a lot of people out there would take your job and think they were the luckiest people in the world!)

If you clash with one or more "difficult" people, make the effort today to find *one* thing you think is good about them—one thing—and be grateful for that.

A very wise friend of mine, Gayle, told me a wonderful story. She was speaking with a young man who was dealing with a "difficult" person at work—someone no one liked or liked working with. My friend told him to see if he could think of one thing good about this person. He thought for some time and finally said, "She looks good in blue." Then Gayle suggested to the young man that he return to work and constantly focus on that good thought; and if he was able, to tell the person what he liked about her.

Several months later, Gayle caught up with the young man and asked him how things were going. With great surprise in his voice he said, "It's amazing. Everything at work has changed. I connect with her much better and she is contributing to the team a lot more and everyone is happier!"

Just one tiny little change like that can transform everything! You can do it! It's your choice.

You will be stunned at how your work life changes when you focus on gratitude and actively look for things for which to be thankful or appreciative. Others will notice the change and, wonder of wonders, you may even find yourself *en-joying* moments of work! (Do you know "enjoy" means *in* joy? You may find yourself being *in joy*.)

Gratitude is *very* powerful!

TUESDAY: **HOME GRATITUDE**

> "What a miserable thing life is: you're living in clover, only the clover isn't good enough."[6]
>
> —Bertolt Brecht

Today is home gratitude day. Find as many things as you can that you are thankful for in your home: your family, your pets, your garden, your plants, your neighbors or community, your teenager's room (there's a challenge!) or that your home is a haven. Be creative! Roam around your home and find as many things as you can. *Make it a family game.* Who can come up with the most things for which to be grateful?

If you hear yourself saying, "I wish I had a new sofa" or "I wish the plumbing were fixed"—catch yourself. Instead say, "I am so thankful we have a sofa and I am saving to have my perfect sofa one day!" Or "at least we *have* water." Or "this roof does not leak and we are warm in cold weather." If your roof *does* leak—then be thankful there are *parts* that do not leak! Remember, you are finding things for which to be thankful, not to complain about. And a complaint is a great opportunity to practice reframing.

There is a wonderful Australian movie called *The Castle,* in which a family who lives at the end of the runway of one of Australia's biggest airports fights to stop their house from being condemned. It is an ugly house on a contaminated block but to this family, it's home. Daryl, the father, makes a very poignant speech about how their house is not a house—it is a home in which love, harmony and joy abound.

It really doesn't matter what your house is like—what's important is how much of a *home* you have created. A home full of love, joy and gratitude is a happy home—even if it needs work.

WEDNESDAY: "THE PAST" GRATITUDE

"Be thankful that you don't already have everything you desire. If you did, what would there be to look forward to?"

—Anonymous

Here is your big chance: Today, your mission—should you choose to accept it—is to work through all the big events in your life that have been negative and reframe them.

Review past relationships, past difficult life circumstances, your parents, siblings, teachers, school, college experiences, friends—anything negative that has happened to you in the past. Now find the gift each of those brought you. How did you grow as a result of each experience? How did your life change as a result of these people or situations? What would you have been like if they had not happened? What opportunities opened up because of them? What did you learn?

Do you now have the ability to let go and move on or to keep going in the face of difficulties? Did those relationships and situations help you know yourself or to grow spiritually? Did they help you decide never be addicted to anything? Did they give you strength of character, the ability to know right from wrong, or the wisdom to not take yourself, or life, so seriously?

What capacities did you develop? Resilience? Strength? Humor? Compassion? Determination? Persistence? Willpower? Courage? Responsibility? Integrity? Ethics? Forgiveness?

These are pretty powerful gifts!

Without those experiences and the choices you made with them, you would not be who you are today. You would not have your unique strengths and areas of potential growth!

Bless those people because they are some of your greatest teachers. Be thankful for the situations because they have helped you grow. The toughest lessons are often the most powerful.

A wonderful book called *Molecules of Emotion* by Candace Pert, the scientist who discovered endorphins, shows us that people who hang onto stuff that has happened to them in life are creating a basis for disease. Some researchers believe forgiveness is a major factor for healing in many cases of back pain.

If you choose not to forgive and let go, or not to find some gratitude in your heart, those things that you cling to from the past can make you bitter, twisted, fearful, angry or disappointed for the rest of your life. They can sit and fester inside you and create the seeds of later disease.

So let go, and find gratitude today!

THURSDAY: **BODY GRATITUDE**

"Grace isn't a little prayer you recite before receiving a meal. It's a way to live."

—Jackie Windspear

Your mission today is to spend the entire day expressing gratitude to your body. You are to say nothing negative, no matter what your stomach, thighs or face look like! Treat your body with respect, give it grace, love it and tell it how thankful you are to it. Be grateful your stomach is digesting your food and bless it today. Be in awe of how well your body works, despite the processed foods, junk foods and sugary drinks you might pour into it!

Be grateful you have hair and if you don't, be grateful you have a head! It's so sad that people only really learn to be grateful for what their bodies are, or do, when they become unwell or disabled in some way.

How often are we grateful for our ability to walk? Not until we can't anymore. When do we value our ability to exercise, move and stretch and how important that is for our body and wellness? Only when we are confined to bed or for some reason cannot move as well as we once did. We treasure how great it is to not have pain once we have lived with pain for a while.

Appreciate the enormous job your body does for you every single moment you are alive. Your faithful body is pumping blood, working hard and bringing you nutrition. Thank it by treating it well from this moment on.

When you have the flu or a cold or a fever, be grateful your immune system is fighting off those germs. Our immune system is working for us every second of every day and yet no one ever says "thank you"! As a gesture of gratitude to your immune system, tell your body, "Today I am going to help you by washing my hands carefully and frequently." Then make sure you do it!

What about your blood and lymph systems? And your nervous system? How do you treat them? Do you know how much your nervous system is battered day to day with stress and yet keeps serving you as best it can?

Stress is a big factor in almost everyone's life—we *must* do activities on a regular basis to bust our stress. Book a massage. Go for a walk. Have a bath and detox your body. Exercise. Rest. Turn off all PDAs, phones and any other electrical thing for 30 minutes every day. Sit in the sun for 20 minutes. Meditate. Laugh. Breathe deeply. Book a yoga or Pilates class. Ask your body what it needs, or ask your heart what your body needs—it will know!

Problems can occur when we don't have rhythm and balance in our lives and we push our body beyond its limits—it tries really, really hard to keep going, but there comes a point when it no longer can. And then we find ourselves with a very serious condition from which we may never recover.

For instance, most of us walk around dehydrated these days. We drink too much coffee, soda and sugary drinks and not enough pure water. By the time we are thirsty, dehydration has already had an effect. This was shown to me dramatically one day in Dallas when I had a dark-field microscopy session. It's an amazing process where we can see our blood's living activity through one drop of blood.

A couple of weeks earlier, I had been thrilled that my red blood cells looked so round and healthy. Then, on the day of the follow-up, it was very hot and I had not been drinking much water. When we looked at my blood—gasp!—the red blood cells were all shriveled up and sad looking! And I hadn't even felt thirsty. I learned that drinking a little bit of good water often was important.

Be kind. Be *very* kind to your body today. It probably works harder for you than anyone or anything else in your life. Bless it, nourish it, say grace over everything you put into it and feel real gratitude for what it does for you.

And on top of *all* that—your body houses your soul. That by itself is worthy of true reverence. (More on that later!)

FRIDAY: **NATURE GRATITUDE**

"To educate yourself for the feeling of gratitude means to take nothing for granted."

—Albert Schweitzer

How many times have you found yourself refreshed, restored and rejuvenated by a walk in the forest, by a stream or beside the ocean? Nature is full of invisible forces working for you all the time to create natural rhythms and currents that affect your entire being and soothe your soul.

Consider sunshine for a minute. Do we stop and thank the sun? Or thank God for the sunshine? Sunshine is the most vital source of vitamin D, which is essential for good health.

What about clean air? It's only when allergy season comes that we realize what a blessing clean air is!

How often do we respect or revere the purity of rain, rivers, snow and other sources of water? Remember, without those, we would all die. There is already a significant shortage of pure drinkable water in the world—appreciate what you have now! Value it and treasure it.

Think of the beauty that surrounds us—the trees, flowers, rainbows, sunsets, sunrises—all of which soothe our souls and feed our bodies essential nutrients. How often do you stop, look around in awe and wonder, and thank everything you see for bringing such beauty and healing to you? We take it all pretty much for granted, don't we?

Be grateful for the winds that clean out the pollution we create. Be grateful for animals that bring us joy, comfort and fascination; the trees that give us shelter; the bees that pollinate the foods we eat; the flowers, plants and herbs that bring us gorgeous scents, colors, tastes and amazing healing; the changing seasons and the spectacular colors of fall; and the endless beauty that surrounds us and fills our hearts.

Without nature, your senses would be very bored!

Even in the concrete jungles we have built, nature has a way of bringing her wisdom to us. Look for the little plants growing out of tiny crevices! Put a plant on your desk at work, or have one inside your home and revere it as your symbol for all nature does for you. Thank the plant, and nature, every day for the oxygen they create and the life forces they bring you.

SATURDAY: HEART GRATITUDE

"It isn't what you have in your pocket that makes you thankful but what you have in your heart."

—Anonymous

Do we really have any idea of the truly immense nature of our hearts?

People think the brain is the most important organ in the body but it's not. The heart rules the rest of the body, and the Institute of Heart Math has scientific evidence of that. (The Institute of Heart Math is a wonderful organization that teaches people how to appreciate their hearts and how to change their lives by paying attention to the heart. Visit www.heartmath.com.)

The heart is *not* just a pump that circulates your blood. Your heart is your world! It's the way you connect to God. Your heart is what connects you to others. It, not your brain, is the seat of your innate intelligence. It is your source of intuition, inspiration, love and life. It is an alchemical vessel.

Today is your day to spend time with your heart. It breaks, it hurts, it feels, it thinks, it constantly sends messages to the rest of your body, orchestrating everything. It is the conductor of a magnificent symphony—you. Yet in our busy, rushed lives, we rarely stop and take time to tune into our heart—to give it a chance to whisper to us.

Bless your heart today. Thank it. Listen *to* it and *through* it. It is very wise, but it often speaks very softly. You have to listen carefully.

If we regularly take time to listen to our heart, we can be aware of a feeling or sense of truly knowing whether something is right or not.

I experienced this on the wedding day of my first marriage. I remember walking down that aisle *knowing* I was doing the wrong thing. Although the marriage did not last, I am grateful for the lessons it taught me.

It has taken me many years to learn to listen to, and through, my heart and I still have a long way to go. Taking courses called "Sacred Service" and "Spirit Healing" (www.spiritualschool.org) has helped me a great deal. Both courses are well worth looking into if you are interested in truly finding your heart, joy and peace and being of service to the world.

Find your heart today. Listen *to* it. Listen *through* it. Bless it. Thank it. Keep talking to it and listening for its guidance in everything.

Today and tomorrow could be the days that change your life!

CHAPTER 2

A WEEK OF **COMPASSION/GRACE**

"Each of us in our own way can try to spread compassion into
people's hearts. Western civilizations these days place great
importance on filling the human 'brain' with knowledge,
but no one seems to care about filling the human 'heart' with
compassion."[1]

—The Dalai Lama

YOUR **SEVEN MINUTES**

How would you define "compassion"? What does it mean to you?

Who are people in your life you would consider compassionate?
Think of a time when someone was compassionate with you. How did
it feel? What did they do or say?

How do you feel when you are compassionate with another? Where
do you feel compassion in your body?

Spend a few moments thinking about times in your life when you
knew you were being selfish. What do you think selfishness does to
compassion?

Reflect on Buddha, Mother Teresa, Christ or any other being that
has lived whom you feel embodies compassion.

Are you compassionate? Could you be more compassionate? Would you *like* to be more of a compassionate person? If so, read on.

AMANDA'S TAKE ON COMPASSION/GRACE

"The whole idea of compassion is based on a keen awareness of the interdependence of all these living beings which are all part of one another and all involved in one another."[2]

—Thomas Merton

My husband Ken and I were talking about compassion and he came up with a definition that resonated with me: Compassion is being compelled, with passion, to take action. That action may be to sit with someone, send them love or hold them in your heart and pray—as long as it involves *doing* something for another person.

I wondered if there was a difference between empathy and compassion. After much deliberation, I decided that empathy allows us to feel what others are feeling—we can sympathize, commiserate or have some sense of understanding—but compassion actually causes us to take action.

Writing this made me recognize another gift my mum gave me—a rare opportunity to experience true empathy and compassion when two of my friends informed me that their mothers were dying. I had already realized that no matter how much we *think* we understand what another person is experiencing when they talk about losing someone they love, we don't really understand until we have gone through something similar. Perhaps it's only then that we can be one with the other person's heart because of our own experience. This is real empathy—where we can step into someone's shoes.

A magical thing had happened after Mum's death, that totally transformed how I related to my friends and taught me more about compassion. I felt my soul was now able to be with another person's soul. As though my heart were their heart. I could just *be* there with them, not doing anything outwardly but *doing* something inwardly—*holding* them and their feelings in my heart. I wanted to do something, even if it was inner activity.

Compassion, to me, is that state where we can somehow see the other person for who they really are and what is going on for them, and we are moved to take action. We really feel what it must be like for the other person to be going through whatever it is they are experiencing, and we want to do something to help them. Although sometimes we have no idea of the other person's life or why we feel this way, we still feel compassion and are moved to do something for them, even if it's just to be kind.

This is a heart-to-heart and spirit-to-spirit connection that is much more powerful than a brain-to-brain one. Compassion is an ongoing activity—a way of living. Compassion transcends time and space!

The phrase, "my heart goes out to you" is common in our culture and it initially led me to think that the seat of compassion was the heart. Apparently, the ancient Egyptians thought the seat of compassion was the liver! They had a hieroglyphic that said "my liver goes out to you."

On reflection, perhaps they're right! The liver deals with all toxicity in our bodies, and many believe negative emotions are stored there. If the liver is blocked with lots of toxic waste, it would keep us from being able to reach out to others. We would be too absorbed with negative emotions and ourselves.

Our hearts (and livers apparently!) actively go out to people through compassion, even if we don't understand why. Our heart gently surrounds those with whom we interact—they feel safe and loved, and if nothing else, they know we are there for them. We don't really have to do anything other than hold them in our hearts because that is doing something. We may need to do more, but this is a start.

With compassion we can often see the larger picture—and we want to help in appropriate ways that still allow the person to experience what they need to, even if it's suffering, in order to make it through their life, learning their lessons. Compassion is healing.

Do you recall the poem about a man who dreams he is walking along a beach with God? As he looks back, he sees that at all the rough times in his life, there is only one set of footprints on the sand. He asks

God, "Why were you not with me at those times?" God answers with love and says, "Those were the times I was carrying you."

Perhaps part of compassion—or most of compassion—is supporting your loved ones and others when they need it most—in whatever way you can.

BEING PRESENT TO THE PERSON AND THE WHOLE

Compassion is a quality that allows God's gifts for us to be exercised. When someone has a desire in their heart to do the right thing but lacks the skills, knowledge or capacity to do it, if we can help, we need to do what we can. Our responsibility is to help others fulfill *their* responsibilities on earth—it's a flow from our responsibilities to theirs and back.

If we remember that:
- ♥ we are all connected through our hearts,
- ♥ we are all part of the whole,
- ♥ we are part of every other living human and they, us,
- ♥ we need to listen to their heart, with our heart, and
- ♥ we need to silence our judgments and listen through our heart to what God is inspiring us to do,

then we can "do unto others as we would have them do unto us."

As author Stephen Covey says in *Seven Habits of Highly Effective People,* "Listen with your eyes for feelings." To really listen to another's heart language, we have to be *absolutely present.* Many people have short attention spans and are often absolutely absent!

Have you ever been talking to someone on the phone and you sense they are distracted? When you hear the keys clicking on their computer keyboard, you *know* it is because they are not really listening to you. How does that make you feel? Have you done this to others?

Do you remember all the content of a conversation when you are only paying attention to it halfheartedly? The center for hearing is in our heads, but we *really* hear with our hearts. If you were listening with your whole being, you would be more respectful and not focus on something else while another person was communicating with you.

Children pick this up very easily. Have you ever had a child say to you, "You're not *listening* to me!" They are experts at knowing when you are there with your whole heart.

Be open, listen carefully and "hear" the other person's heart (with your heart's "ears"). *Be* with them. Remember the hologram: you two are really a part of each other and a part of everything. Offer absolute presence, love, support, grace, tenderness and more love. I think that is part of compassion. And it's not so easy. I wish I did it a *lot* better. But I am doing the best I can—which is what we are all doing.

My friend Mary is one of the most compassionate people I know. I am convinced Mama brought Mary to me to heal me of Lyme disease and to become my soul sister. She is an amazing single mother of three children, one of whom is autistic. Her life is committed to those children, and through very difficult circumstances, she has remained one of the kindest, most loving people I have ever come to know.

Her heart includes everyone—no matter who they are or what they do—and she seems to find a way to connect with every heart and spirit she meets. Mary perceives every person as a reflection of God on earth and works at helping them do what God sent them to do. She always tries to empower people and has a great capacity for discernment. Through inspiration, Mary, a very godly person, a master herbalist and a master dowser, seems to know in her heart the truth about others—who they really are, and the perfect thing to do to help them.

Even if others are not behaving in the best way, Mary finds compassion for them, although she doesn't make excuses for or allow unacceptable behavior. She seems very wise, soft and kind, yet incredibly strong, with integrity, all at once. When I listen to the tone of her voice, I can really *feel* her caring and compassion coming through.

Mary even taught me how to pray. The first time I heard her say a prayer, I thought, "*Now* I know how to pray." Although I had not really thought about how I talked to God, the way Mary did it was so beautiful and full of love and compassion for others that I knew what

I had been doing was not really praying; it was just asking for stuff and occasionally thanking God.

I feel blessed to have met Mary—she has saved my life in many ways. I believe I am much more "present" with God now when I pray. Plus, with prayer and inspiration, Mary finds ways to cure almost anything! Thank you, Mary!

So what are the little steps that might lead each of us closer to living a life of compassion?

The more I research and write, the more I realize the essence of compassion is connection—connecting our head with our heart; connecting our heart to the heavens; connecting our heart with other people's hearts; and all being connected with a "giant world heart."

Compassion shines from the heart, along with love, kindness, acceptance, tenderness, caring, forgiveness and grace—many of the qualities we associate with God. I am convinced that the heart is the organ through which God connects to us, and connects to others *through* us, and therefore, connects us to them. The heart connection is alchemical in that it can transform everything.

SELF-CENTEREDNESS IS SEPARATION

> "The purpose of life is not to be happy. It is to be useful, to be honorable, to be compassionate, to have it make some difference that you have lived and lived well."
>
> —Ralph Waldo Emerson

After much deliberating, I have concluded that compassion is the opposite of selfishness or self-centeredness. We cannot be compassionate and thinking only of ourselves at the same time.

In my research, a frequent theme for compassion was recognizing we are all part of the whole and we are not separate. When we are self-centered—that is, when we are the center of our own little universe and our whole universe at the same time—we lose our awareness of our connection and responsibility to the rest of humanity, the world and the cosmos.

Sometimes we are self-centered in some areas of our lives and not others, or with some people and not others. Selfishness is essentially a state of unconscious separation. It is unusual to be in a state of compassion and be selfish at the same time!

Compassion requires us to focus outwards towards others and to have a consciousness of the whole. When we are self-absorbed, our focus is on ourselves and we are totally asleep to spiritual currents swirling around us and the millions of other feeling souls.

Many people are wondering about their purpose in life, saying "There must be more to life than this." Modern lifestyles seem to discourage heart connection although we appear to be more electronically connected than ever.

Serving others and acting through compassion and inspiration gives us a sense of purpose.

Realizing that there is no separation between any of us is the antidote to *self-centered*-ness. We *are* all one. We are never really isolated or completely separate from others or God. We are all affected by the same influences—the moon, sun and sea and the rhythms of the earth and cosmos.

Once we realize we *are* all connected and what we do *will* affect everyone and everything else, how can we demand conditions that are for our sole benefit, ignoring, or not caring about, the effect on others?

By separating ourselves from God and others, and wanting only what *we* desire to satisfy our *own* emotions, wants or needs, we create misery for ourselves and others. In selfish mode, we cannot be in our hearts and connected. We are caught in negative emotions triggered by thoughts of "What about *me*? What about *my* feelings? How dare they do that to *me*?" (As if "they" were terrible beings outside of us, and not a part of us!)

These *self*-orientated thoughts create negative emotions of anger, jealousy, resentment, bitterness and disappointment that keep us separated from our own hearts, let alone anyone else's.

The Dalai Lama, one of the masters of compassion, says, "If you want others to be happy, practice compassion. If you want to be happy, practice compassion."

If you are not feeling joyful, have a long look at yourself—are you in selfish mode? If so, go out immediately, focus outwards, seek to serve and do something self-*less* and be full of compassion for someone else!

GRACE

Compassion is also about grace—God's grace and allowing His grace to flow through us. That means not condemning others, giving up on them or judging them.

I am not sure we can give anything like God's grace but we can let His flow through us to others. God pours His grace out on us. We are forgiven, blessed and loved continuously. We are given endless, unlimited grace from God and we usually remain totally oblivious to it. Our work is to become conscious of grace and pass it on—even if others don't appear to deserve it!

We can share grace by being gracious, as well as being forgiving and loving. We can also give someone the benefit of the doubt; assume the best about them; be compassionate instead of "right"; say nothing when we could criticize; speak only positively; think only good thoughts about another; put them in our heart; help them if they need it; and choose not to take offense.

Choose to give grace to others. It takes a lot to continually forgive, bless and love, but it would be a great goal, wouldn't it? Even if it took a lifetime! It could be something we decide to do each day—to give grace. Make it a morning mantra: "Today I will be gracious, forgive, bless and love everyone."

As you read this, I can hear you thinking, "Be realistic!"

Well, how about, "Today I will forgive, bless and love as many people as I can"? Or be specific each day, and rotate through "my husband/wife/children/parents/friends/siblings." Or start with baby steps—"Today, I will give my partner the benefit of the doubt all day *and* I will choose to be kind rather than right."

UNCONDITIONAL LOVE AND TENDERNESS

"Be kinder than necessary. Everyone you meet is fighting a hard battle."

—Philo of Alexandria

Real unconditional love and tenderness are components of compassion. When I think about tenderness, I imagine the way we hold a tiny, fragile, delicate item or the way a loving parent looks at their child. Our physical movements, eyes and voice tones convey tenderness. In a gesture of tenderness, love pours forth from the heart, and is expressed to others in many ways.

Are you so stressed and rushed in life that you grasp life, people and things with a tension-filled, vice-like grip? Do you unknowingly squeeze hard and harm or crush what is in your hands? Or do you hold your life and loved ones as if they were precious—and treasure them by being tender, loving and gentle?

Someone who had seen me speak years ago sent a wonderful email—he was talking of the value of "dropping to his heart" before he connects with someone he cares about:

"When I am sharing with someone I care for and the question arises, 'HOW do I drop down to my heart?' I simply share that it all starts with the tone . . . I feel what is in my heart and I express it ever so gently . . . my voice actually lowers and softens . . . all unconsciously by the way . . . and I know I am in my heart!"

It's so easy to be thoughtless and heartless, to judge and be direct or harsh. That is what happens when we react rather than respond. If we can just take a second, drop to our hearts and respond *from* our hearts, we are more conscious and tender and make better choices. True strength comes from the gentle wisdom of the heart.

Listen to your voice tones—they are the key indicator of how much tenderness is present. Be aware of how your eyes feel; we can "feel" tenderness in our eyes. And last but not least, notice your hand gestures. I have watched parents who touch their babies in such a tender way that tears come to my eyes; and lovers who touch the cheek of their partner in a way that conveys more love than any words could. A tender gesture is very powerful.

These four components—*self-less*-ness, grace, love and tenderness—seem to work together in my heart to bring me closer to living life with compassion for myself and others.

As always, compassion is a choice. We can choose to *want* to be more compassionate and more conscious of compassionate behavior, and then *be* more compassionate by practicing.

Here is a week's worth of practice!

DAILY SCHEDULE

SUNDAY AND MONDAY: SELF-LESS-NESS

"In separateness lies the world's great misery; in compassion lies the world's great strength."

—Buddha

This is a two-day exercise. For two days, try to focus only on others and how you might help, support and bless them and allow God's grace to flow through you to them.

These two days are not about you at *all*. Not even a teeny bit! They are all about you doing something for others—being in the activity of compassion and serving others with love, kindness and tenderness.

Do something for a family member that you know will delight them. Do a chore that is not yours just to save the other person from having to do it. Do volunteer work. Help your neighbor or community. Pay the toll for the person behind you. Find an old person living alone and do some manual labor for them, or better—do it *and* then spend some time visiting with them. There are a million things you can do to focus on and help others!

The purpose of these activities is for you to not think of yourself and your wants for *two whole days*. The more difficult you find it, the more interesting you might find the results!

Remember to do all of this with a heart full of compassion and caring for others, which means your intentions are sincere and pure. If you do it just to have others say what a saint you are, then it won't work!

Perhaps a mantra these two days could be, "Can I do something to help you?" If they say "no," send them love—that is doing a lot!

You may be surprised to see how different the world appears during and after these two days, and how many people are affected and how your interactions with them seem to change.

TUESDAY: COMPASSION FOR YOUR BOSS, COLLEAGUES AND CUSTOMERS

You can transform every aspect of your work (and life) with compassion.

Imagine what life would be like if we actually encountered customer-service people who had compassion for our suffering. I know my best experiences have been when I *have felt* someone genuinely does care that I am frustrated, upset or disappointed rather than simply saying "I'm sorry you're having these problems."

Compassion transforms customer service.

Imagine too what life would be like if you had compassion for your colleagues—even if prior to now, you have judged them idiots. Give them some grace! People may be confused, stressed, overloaded, have a difficult situation at home, not be trained well or have a hundred other reasons for not performing the way you think they should. Compassion can transform your relationships with colleagues.

The best bosses I have ever had are those who really showed me compassion. They knew I had plenty of areas where I needed growth, but they still believed in me. They treated me with understanding and kindness when I made mistakes, and they worked with me to help me learn and supported me. I felt good about myself around them. If you are a boss—do you think the people that you lead feel the way I did? Compassion transforms leadership.

Maybe your life would change if you viewed everyone at work through a compassionate heart and treated them that way! Maybe they would miraculously turn into great colleagues and bosses and they would wonder what kind of personality transplant *you* had undergone! Your mission this day is to be compassionate with everyone at work.

♥ Be selfless—focus outward and not towards yourself, sincerely offer to help people and be understanding. If you see someone stressed and rushed, find a way to help them.

♥ Be gracious—pass God's grace onto as many people as you can. Be patient, kind, tolerant, forgive them, give them the benefit of the doubt and just be kind!

♥ Try your best to unconditionally love (or accept) them as they are.

♥ Be tender with them. See them through tender eyes. Be kind again! And again! And always be gentle with them—and yourself.

WEDNESDAY AND THURSDAY: COMPASSION AT HOME

"The Lord is full of compassion and gracious, slow to anger, and plenteous in mercy."

—Psalms 103:8

Okay, these are the easier days. This activity is so important and there are so many people involved that you have two days to practice.

It's easy to have compassion for our children. We give them endless space to be who they are, faults and all!

But do we do that with our partners? Siblings? Relatives? We are more likely to give compassion to our friends than to any of our relatives, or our partners! And yet, it is our partners who are our greatest teachers in life. They volunteered—though maybe not consciously—to help us grow and develop emotionally and spiritually. Find it in your heart to have compassion for them—*you* may not be an easy task!

I know my husband deserves a medal of valor and a lot of compassion for the life he has with me! I obviously had a *lot* of lessons to learn, and he is doing a great job in spite of difficult circumstances. I need to remind myself of that more often!

When we are self-orientated, we see our partner as the problem. We don't even know we are projecting onto them all of our "stuff" and not really seeing their heart. We see the image that we have created based on *our* past—not the truth of who they are.

When we are compassionate, we understand they have taken on a *big* task and that without our partners, we might be stagnating. We find gratitude for them and their gift. We understand the challenge they face with us and have a sense of the difficulties they experience as they help us grow.

Teenagers deserve compassion, as they may be the greatest teachers of all. Try to remember what it was like when you had hormones coursing through your body and you loved and hated your parents at the same time. It's amazing how we are seen as brilliant by our toddlers who want to be around us all the time, yet those same toddlers grow into teenagers who avoid us like the plague and think we are embarrassing, controlling and total morons! Our work is to love them, discipline them and teach them with compassion, despite what they think of us! It's not easy, but someone has to do it and that someone would be you!

Remember that compassion is a blend of forgiveness, self-less-ness, unconditional love, grace and tenderness. And at times, it requires us to be firm.

Teenagers, too, need to have compassion for you and the *huge* job you have taken on with them—but we are more grown-up than them, so it's more our responsibility.

These two days are all about constantly forgiving and focusing on others' needs, giving everyone at home as much grace as you can—*especially when they don't deserve it*, loving and accepting everyone *as they are* (a big one for most of us), and being as tender as you can with them.

Look for the habitual patterns of behavior you have adopted in your family and re-pattern them to include compassion. Think of these patterns as simply cast in sand—awaiting new impressions to be pressed onto them. A good or blessed pattern will change everything.

If you can't manage any of the above, then work on having a tender voice—show your love and compassion through your voice all day!

FRIDAY: COMPASSION FOR YOUR "ENEMIES"

"Compassion compels us to reach out to all living beings, including our so-called enemies, those people who upset or hurt us. Irrespective of what they do to you, if you remember that all beings like you are only trying to be happy, you will find it much easier to develop compassion towards them. The true aim of cultivation of compassion is to develop the courage to think of others and to do something for them."[3]

—The Dalai Lama

The above quote from the Dalai Lama pretty much says it all. Can you find the courage in your heart to think of others and do something today to help your "enemy"?

The concept of enemy is pretty foreign to me because unless we are at war, our day-to-day life is not usually full of enemies. However, we often have people who have hurt us, who annoy us, humiliate us, frighten us, shout at us, belittle us, are unkind to us, offend us, or cause us difficulty, frustration, disappointment and pain, or are simply "mean" to us.

These are the "enemies" that we need to have the courage to forgive and see if we can help in some way. If we can't love them, then at least we can hold them in our hearts for some time, so our hearts can work miracles together, and try to think kindly of them. This takes courage and "will forces"—a conscious act of will to do something that does not feel "natural." If you practice, it will soon feel natural—and great!

If the concept of actually helping these so-called enemies is too much of a first step for you, then maybe you can think of this person or people in a way that is neutral rather than negative. From neutral, you can move to thinking something kind or good about them. Do they look good in blue? Then you can try understanding how unhappy they may be to behave the way they do, or how difficult life must be for them. Move to feeling for them in your heart, and from there you will be closer to compassion.

This may take a little longer than one day—but start today! You'll be surprised at who benefits the most.

SATURDAY: **COMPASSION FOR YOURSELF**

"If you have no compassion for yourself, then you are not capable of developing compassion for others."

—The Dalai Lama

Reflect all day today on "What compassion do I give myself?"

Many people judge themselves harshly. Do you allow God's grace to flow through and to you for the mistakes you make? Or do you beat yourself up as a failure? Mistakes bring learning. If you've never made a mistake, you've missed a lot of learning opportunities. Some of our biggest and most beneficial lessons (which do not seem so beneficial at the time) come from our biggest "mistakes."

Imagine what a toddler learning to walk would do if every time he or she fell down, we shouted at them, told them what silly idiots they were and used the kind of phrases we use on ourselves all the time. Pretty soon, they would cry and not attempt to walk anymore.

We limit ourselves in the same way when we give ourselves no graciousness, mercy or compassion. Are you hard on yourself? Do you drive yourself mercilessly? Do you think you are "ridiculous," or do you talk to yourself in the tone of voice that says, "I am an idiot"?

Do you deny any feelings you have and just swallow what happens to you and never allow yourself to feel pain? Do you load yourself with guilt or accept others dumping *all* the blame on you and not accepting any themselves? If so, stop doing this today!

We are all human, doing the best we can, and we need to give *ourselves* a *lot* of grace and compassion.

Today, your task is to be endlessly tender and loving with yourself. Be gracious to yourself for things you have done in the past and move on. Allow yourself to feel some of the pain that may have been suppressed for a long time. It really is okay to feel the pain—as long as it comes out and you deal with yourself compassionately. (Best you do that with someone you trust and when you have time to cry.) Give yourself permission to feel whatever your heart needs to. Recognize and release stuff that is held inside and blocking your progress.

Set the intention before you climb out of bed: "Today I will be compassionate (loving, tender and grace-giving) with myself. I will pay attention to my *true* self, the one that lives in my heart, and not the selfish, spoiled personality (which is the "front" I put on for the world to supposedly keep me safe)."

Your heart will rule whatever you say to yourself and how you treat yourself today. That judgmental, nasty, critical, nagging voice will be silent—all day and hopefully for a lot longer! You have been doing the best you can with what you've had, so pat yourself on the back and give yourself a *TA-DA!*

You will be gentle and kind to yourself as you "learn how to walk" again—this time on the path of compassion.

CHAPTER 3

A WEEK OF **HOPE**

"If you lose wealth, you lose nothing.
If you lose health, you lose something.
If you lose hope, you lose everything."

—Mr. Gojani, a refugee from Kosovo, describing
his family's journey out of their country

YOUR **SEVEN MINUTES**

This week our focus is on hope.

Can you think of situations in life where you were full of hope? How did you feel and act? How did you treat others?

At other times, when you felt hopeless or uncertain, how did you behave and feel?

Recall times when you were driven by fear instead of hope. What outcome did you experience when fear was in control? What is the difference in how you felt, acted and treated others when hope was your guide?

Recall what you said to yourself when hope was your companion and compare that with a time when fear ruled your thoughts. Which made you feel stressed and heavy? Which made you feel more relaxed and light?

What happens in your life when you have hopeful expectations?

AMANDA'S TAKE ON HOPE

"But we also exult in our tribulations, knowing that tribulation brings about perseverance; and perseverance, proven character; and proven character, hope; and hope does not disappoint."

—Romans 5: 3-5

RESILIENCE

Having been a mostly resilient, optimistic person the majority of my life, I am blessed with taking the *hope road* most of the time. I am convinced that there *is* hope in all situations and that most things happen for a reason. I busy myself with finding a way through the circumstances rather than giving up and feeling hopeless.

I was blessed with a couple of great friends who held my hand when I lost all my money at the age of 45. I am so grateful to Julianna, Evan and Christine for their love and support—and the hope and courage they gave me. With that support, I could recover and continue when everything looked bleak.

If you are going through a difficult experience, seek out people who are optimistic and hopeful; avoid those who are full of doom and gloom. Negative people can destroy your spirit and your ability to be resilient and persevere.

Sometimes though, negative people can make us stronger. They force us to develop our strength of character and be all we can be, if we don't succumb to their negativity or hopelessness. Many really positive, resilient people came from backgrounds where their families or circumstances seemed hopeless, yet they made a decision early on that they would never be like that. See—there's a reason for everything!

If the world seems full of negative people to you, it's time to review how you actually perceive the world. I realized this one day when I was in my twenties and I was overwhelmed with how many problems everyone I met was having—or that's the way it seemed. I never seemed to meet people who were happy—until I had a blinding flash of the obvious! I suddenly recognized that I was basically asking people with my spirit and nonverbals, "What is wrong with your life?"

I would dwell on what was going wrong rather than what was right and wonderful in my own life. Once I had that "aha" moment, my life changed and so did everybody else's! Suddenly there were all these happy people around me. It was an unforgettable lesson and gift!

Resilience is a quality that is very useful for every aspect of our lives. We can't be great salespeople without resilience—or leaders, parents, friends or spouses/partners. With resilience, we can make mistakes and learn rather than see ourselves as failures.

The seed of resilience lies in hope. An Eastern proverb tells us to "fall down seven times, get up eight!" That is resilience. *Smart* resilience is when we learn from each fall and rise wiser and able to deal with the next challenge (which may be a life-changing wake-up call) in a different way. It's difficult to have resilience without hope or the courage hope gives us.

A woman I recently spoke to described her very difficult situation. Her father had died two months previously; her mother was not doing well as a result; her own job was in jeopardy; one daughter had post-partum depression; another daughter with a mental illness announced she was pregnant; and her third child was diagnosed with a brain tumor. Needless to say, she was exhausted and very stressed.

Although she was feeling overwhelmed and it seemed that not much else could go wrong, she had hope and faith, which gave her the resilience to keep going. She had more than the faith that God would give her the strength she needed; she had the will to hold that faith despite what happened. She had faith in herself that she could continue to not just cope but also handle the situations with equanimity. She believed—and often reminded herself—that good would somehow emerge from these seemingly endless crises, and she *chose* to remain hopeful.

How resilient are you? If you don't seem to have much bounce-back ability, you might need to focus on developing hope and faith by hanging around people who have a lot of it. These people can help as they light your candles of hope and faith.

Choose to monitor and change your language, and your thinking, where necessary. Catch yourself repeating negative and hopeless phrases in your head. Read inspirational stories of hope and faith and how they have helped others.

These are just some of the many activities—notice they are *activities*, since they require some *action* on your part—that can build your hope, faith and resilience.

COURAGE AND HOPE VS. FEAR

"We can easily forgive a child who is afraid of the dark; the real tragedy of life is when men are afraid of the light."

—Plato

For me, it seems that the polar opposite of hope is fear. We travel between the two poles, but if we don't make a conscious effort to spend most of our time at the hope end, we will unconsciously live in fear that blocks life forces and joy.

Hopelessness is often triggered by a fear of something—perhaps a fear of failure. Or a fear of losing something, someone or some battle. Or a fear that whatever we are facing is so large we cannot conquer it. There are many fears ready to grip us at any time. We have to be vigilant!

As a little girl, for some reason I don't understand, I was afraid of the dark. I was particularly afraid of scary monsters that lived under my bed. I would lie in bed fearful and sweating until hopelessness set in. I let my fear become so overpowering that I gave in to hopelessness. It was always amazing to me that as soon as the light was turned on, the room was safe again. Most of our fears are like that—they dissolve when light is shone onto, or into, them.

God's love is the light that guides you from fear to hope. He is always shining that light for us. When all appears dark, we aren't aware that we have closed our eyes! Hope acts like a candle in a dark room; it lights up our surroundings and shines into the future, showing us the way and dispelling the fears that create obstacles on our path.

Patience must go hand in hand with hope! Many times we need to wait for God's timing—although we want what we want *now*, or for things to be fixed or relationships healed immediately. Often, that is not what would be best for everyone involved! We need to wait patiently for God with a heart full of hope. It takes effort, persistence and work to do this.

How do we develop the capacity to be open to the light and hope God gives us?

First, look around you! Everywhere we look, there are miracles that unfold each day—whether it's the flowers blooming, babies being born, seasons changing, or the body working every minute in amazing ways.

Second, look back on your life and remember some event that seemed terrible at the time, and how it miraculously turned out months or years later to be the best thing that could have happened to you.

Third, listen to your heart. Recall all those times in life when you have felt some kind of guidance. People hear God differently—as a booming voice, a feeling of heat or fire, a burning in the heart. You may hear a clear, distinct "voice from your heart" giving you wisdom, or a whisper that tells you something you *know* is the right thing to do. It may even be a clear thought without words. Remember a time when you were in crisis and prayed, and things worked out from there. This is how you tap into your heart's "knowing"—by listening.

Fourth, ask. Ask for God to be so clear in your life that you know it is Him; so clear that there is no way you can doubt His presence or influence.

Fifth, pray. Pray for your heart to guide you and show you the truth. Pray about everything you do, and be thankful for everything that happens. With God's help, things will always work out for the good.

In Proverbs 23:7, we are told, "As a man thinketh in his heart, so is he." Fear disappears when we have clear thinking in our hearts. By clear thinking, I mean that we know exactly what we are hearing, seeing and supposed to be doing.

Imagine there is an ongoing battle between light and dark in the heart. If we clearly choose and focus on the light, the fear or darkness disappears as the light rays shine through us and we shine the light on our darkness. If we can consciously operate from the light in our hearts, then fear will never grip us again—or not for long, anyway. When we use our heart's "knowing" to guide us, we are filled with hopeful expectations.

If you are feeling fear, know clearly (or seek) what God wants from you, and press on anyway. Do it with an attitude of, "So there, take *that,* fear!"

HOPE AND HEALTH

"Hope deferred makes the heart sick, but when longing is fulfilled, it is a tree of life."

—Proverbs 13:12

Many studies have shown that optimism and hope play a vital part in the healing process. How people view a diagnosis or their situation can determine whether they live or die. People who are full of faith and hope are often those who have "miraculous" cures.

Being full of hope makes us seem vibrant, colorful and alive. Hope increases our life force through physical and spiritual breathing. It strengthens every cell in the body and heals us.

Have you ever noticed that when we are fearful or stressed, our breathing stops? In moments of fear, we gasp, freeze, take shallow breaths and lose the capacity to move, listen or hear. Why do we say "paralyzed by fear"? Because fear instantly stops our life force.

What a doctor or any health or complementary practitioner says when we are ill must be very carefully considered. The health professional must allow some place for hope in the patient's heart. Remember that a heart filled with hope can transmute everything.

If we suffer from a serious illness, who knows that a new cure will not be found next week? Who knows if a miracle will occur? Who knows what a prayer can do? Who knows if there is someone healing this condition in another country? God does! And your job is to have faith that if you are meant to find this cure, you will—so go look!

And if you feel a particular healthcare practitioner has little hope for you, it is critical you find one who shares your hopeful heart. No person is God. They cannot give you a sentence! They can tell you what they find and what they have learned to date, but that's all they really know at that time. Who knows what experiences *other* people have had that would transform your attitude to one of confidence and hope?

Never give up. Hope and faith may be the only things needed to keep you alive and make you well, or to allow you to follow whatever *your* path is—whether it involves healing or not—with peace and equanimity.

LEARNED HOPE IS A CHOICE—IT TAKES WORK

"There are no hopeless situations, only people who are hopeless about them."

—Anonymous

What's the difference between people who give up on a situation because it's "hopeless" and those who try and try again? The difference is persistence, resilience, hope and what those people say to themselves. Some of us don't realize we have old patterns and habits of negativity that leave us depressed, fearful, un-motivated, helpless and hopeless.

When we fall into the trap of being victims, we give up all responsibility for ourselves and cannot see how we have contributed to our circumstances. Many times we blame others or find excuses, such as "I couldn't help it," "It's not my fault" and "There was nothing I could do."

There is often no truth in these kinds of statements. We always have a choice. God gave us free will—which means we have a choice in how we behave, respond to something or deal with something. Sometimes it's hard for us to hear this and we resist—because it means we have to take responsibility for what happens and how we respond. It means we have to stop blaming.

We are never alone; there is a spiritual world full of angels who are always sitting beside us, waiting to help, *but we need to ask!* Things are *never* hopeless while the angels are there, and they are always there in some form—even after fear blocks our breathing.

Stop saying negative things to yourself about any situation, and tell yourself, "I can do all things in He who strengthens me." When you feel negative or hopeless, take some time and focus your attention on your heart area and, if possible, connect with your spiritual "helpers." You may feel peace and hope, and your body may relax.

Have you noticed that one of the words used to describe hopelessness, or the state where one loses the will to keep going, is "disheartened"? In this state, we have disconnected from our hearts. If we make the effort to reconnect with, and operate from, clarity in our hearts, we are choosing hope.

Heart clarity expands us; it connects us with the spiritual realms; it gives us courage; it works together with faith; it heals; and it builds.

Fear stops life forces from flowing, separates us from God, paralyzes us and is the basis of almost all negative emotions—anger, jealousy, disappointment, lack of self esteem, thoughts of inadequacy, cowardice, and frustration, to name only a few. Anytime you have a negative emotion, stop and ask yourself, "What am I frightened of here? What fear is behind this behavior/thinking/response?"

These are extremely powerful questions that can transform a situation by shining a light on the fears that lurk in the dark, controlling our moods and behaviors without our knowing.

Keep asking the questions until you have shone the light of hope into every little nook and cranny of your being.

Eliminate fearful self-talk and replace it with hopeful inspiration!

WHERE DO YOU FEEL HOPE?

We know hope grows in the heart, but it takes work to be able to identify *where* in the body hope is felt.

Recall a situation in which you were really hopeful, or at least had *some* hope for a positive outcome. How did you feel? Were you aware of any physical sensations? How did you breathe?

You probably felt really alive because hope is linked to life force and the breath. What did your voice sound like? How much energy did you have? Maybe you felt light, or your world actually looked brighter. Or was there a sense of peace? Maybe you felt calmer. Make sure that the next time you feel full of hope you pay special attention to finding the place where you feel it in your body.

Do you have actual physical reactions to fear? Most people do, although we are mostly unconscious of it. Does fear "grip" you or do you have a "sinking" feeling in the pit of your stomach or feel heaviness somewhere? Do you clench your jaws, grind your teeth, have trouble sleeping, have diarrhea, have neck or back pain, lose your ability to focus, become confused, angry and aggressive? Or do you become hyperalert? The list could be endless.

If you can identify the bodily sensation of fear, then you can recognize it, shine light on it, and by identifying it for what it really is, make it evaporate! Well, maybe it doesn't exactly evaporate, but you at least will be conscious of the real issue.

Focus on the difference between where you feel fear and where you feel hope. The more you can differentiate, the more awareness you will have and the more consciously you can choose how you wish to think and feel.

It always *seems* easier to let fear rule the day. We can hide, succumb, be the victim, be hopeless or take no action. It may *seem* easier, but it is not the way to be truly alive and joyful.

We need to know that God is beside us and have the faith, strength and courage to stand up (with His help) and face our fears. We need to move away from what is causing those fears, or challenge them and fill ourselves with hope instead. But we need to *do something*, and to *be conscious* of when we are being driven by fear!

A clear heart will always show us the path of hope. Our fears mostly focus on caution, hazards, problems and danger. A balance between the two stops us from doing dangerous or silly things. But allowing fear to dominate our thinking stops us from feeling alive.

Hope is always available to us. So are our spiritual helpers! If we choose to ask for help, look for and focus on hope, fear dissipates. Just believing hope exists can increase it!

Hope can give us courage, persistence, willpower, resilience, strength and joy. Hopelessness takes them away.

Why *do* people respond so differently to similar situations? Because of the choices they make, the way they look at things, how they pre-program themselves, old patterns and habits, and how much life force they have. Focusing on our breathing—especially our "spiritual" breath (imagine you are breathing in light and love with each breath)—can help reprogram our old patterns by increasing our life forces.

There is always hope. *Always*. No matter how bad things seem, if you seek God's direction and wait, the sun returns. Things pass. Time heals. Joy comes back, even after tragedies of monumental proportions.

DAILY SCHEDULE

SUNDAY: HOPE AND FAITH

"Hoping does not mean doing nothing. It means going about
our assigned tasks, confident that God will provide the meaning
and the conclusion. It means a confident, alert expectation that
God will do what He said He will do. It is imagination put in the
harness of faith. It is a willingness to let God do it in His way and
in His time. It is the opposite of making plans that we demand
God put into effect, telling Him both how and when to do it."[1]

—Eugene H. Peterson

Today is your day for putting your faith in something bigger than you! It doesn't matter whether you call that entity God, Love, Buddha, Allah, Universe, Spirit, the Divine or Spiritual Wisdom, as long as it has meaning for you!

As you go through all your tasks today, recognize there is a much larger world than you can see. Try to sense the spiritual nature of the world. See and feel how full of hope things really are. There *is vast spiritual wisdom in action here.*

Check to see you are doing your part in your life responsibly. Look for the hope and light inside what appears dark, and if you can't find the light, hold onto faith or pray that it will come. Allow the future to unfold without pushing or needing or wanting what you want to happen now!

Put your faith in the fact that someday, you might understand the "grand plan" of your life. You will see that many outcomes that you may have thought were the worst in the world, turned out to be the best.

Perhaps a relationship breaks down and you separate. At the time, you are crushed. You feel no hope. You can't go on. Of course you can and you do! And with hindsight, you look back and thank God for the blessings.

For example, if your previous relationship had not ended, you would never have met the real man or woman of your dreams! Or you may not have made the trip of a lifetime. Or you might eventually realize that the person you so adored had a lot more baggage than you realized, and you were actualy lucky to escape when you did!

Who knows what the disabled, troubled or difficult child brings as their gifts. Our friend Mary's son was diagnosed with severe autism. She was told there was nothing to be done and there was no hope. That wasn't the right thing to say to Mary!

As a result of the gifts from her son Michael, Mary has discovered both her incredible capacity to heal and the many treatments that have helped hundreds of people that were never used before for autism or other health issues. Mary's life has not been easy and still is not easy. But she does her work cheerfully and diligently, and makes the effort to help Michael and others heal. She believes and has absolute faith that he will be healed. She has fought and continues to fight with amazing courage to make things better for him. She makes things happen when she is told it is impossible. Nothing takes away her faith and hope.

This is a shared story of many courageous parents who maintain hope in the face of seemingly insurmountable problems. And every parent who has fought this battle will tell you that the gifts and joy their child has brought them are immeasurable.

We don't know what the future holds and I don't think we are meant to, because that takes away the element of mystery and the lesson and discipline of faith and hope.

Our lessons may not be learned if we don't experience some suffering, pain, loss, sorrow or uncertainty. If we are never uncertain, fearful or confused, faith and hope are not practiced. And we need to practice them—they are like muscles. Use them or lose them!

Every moment, exercise your hope and faith that the spiritual world exists—that God makes good out of bad and brings light into the darkness. Actively hold that hope in your heart—it is required for the transmutation in the alchemical process happening in your heart.

MONDAY: FIND WHERE HOPE LIVES IN YOUR BODY

> "If you lose hope, somehow you lose the vitality that keeps life moving, you lose that courage to be, that quality that helps you go on in spite of it all."
>
> —Martin Luther King, Jr.

Today is the day for you to clearly find where hope lives in your body!

Find a place where you can sit uninterrupted for a while. Take a few deep breaths and then, as vividly as you can, recall and then "relive" a situation where things did not look good and you were driven by fear. (Pick a moderate fear scenario, not a terrifying one!) What did you feel and where did you feel it?

Now think of another challenging situation where you were hope-filled. What were the sensations in your body?

Write down the differences between the two memories as clearly, and as descriptively, as you can. Describe the physical sensations; what your feelings were; where you felt them in your body; what they were like; how you behaved; and how others responded to you.

How connected did you feel to God or the spiritual realms in both conditions? Write down anything you can think of that was different between the two situations.

Once you are conscious of the differences, you can be more aware of the polarity—hope or fear—from which you are operating at any time. And if you find yourself at the fear and darkness end, move towards hope and light.

This reminds me of the brightness or contrast bar in a computer. As we move the cursor towards one end of the bar, the screen image and all we see lightens or darkens. As we slide up and down the hope/fear continuum, our whole world lightens as we move to hope, and darkens the closer we travel to fear.

Write notes to yourself at home and at work that say "Hope!" to remind you to choose hope and faith, and not fear or hopelessness. Put one on your desk or in your drawer as a reminder and maybe even on your mobile phone! Or put one on the wall of your bedroom so it's the first thing you see in the morning.

These notes may sound silly but they work as symbols to remind us that we can choose hope any time we have the courage and will to do it.

Go to bed re-creating that feeling of hope inside you.

TUESDAY: HOPE FOR YOURSELF

"Consult not your fears but your hopes and your dreams. Think not about your frustrations but about your unfulfilled potential. Concern yourself not with what you tried and failed in but with what it is still possible for you to do."

—Pope John XXIII

We all make mistakes. We are all constantly learning how to do things better and doing the best we can with what we have.

These are not new ideas, of course, but we would think they were if we watched how most people treat themselves. I bet you would never say to your best friend (or even your enemies) the sorts of things you say to yourself.

There are times in life when you may be in a very difficult situation that you cannot escape from or change immediately, but you can still have courage, consciousness, a plan, a dream and a hope to remove yourself.

If you choose to operate with hope, everything changes. It's magical, but then anytime you consciously bring God or light into your life, it's magical.

Look at yourself with *hope-full* eyes. You *will* lose weight. You *do* have the strength to do this (whatever "this" is). Things *will* improve. Things may not change in the time frame in which *you* want them to, because God may have another, much better plan for you. So be patient. And wait with a heart full of hope.

Think of all the aspects of your life and/or body with which you are unhappy or disappointed, such as your weight, appearance, smoking, addictions, finances and relationships. Examine how you view these things and what you say to yourself about them. Are you using fear-based judgments or hope-full thinking?

A hope-filled heart will give you strength and courage to continue the journey. (If your concern is an abusive relationship, be honest about the reality of things changing and seek help wherever you can.)

Perhaps if you are at the "hope pole," you won't be driven to eat so much. Perhaps, just perhaps, fear was driving you to eat. Or if you have hope, you won't fight as much or feel so maligned in relationships and life. Or with hope, you will have the courage and strength to give up smoking/drinking/addiction. Who knows what miracles will happen when you operate from hope!

Wait patiently, with positive expectations. Take the right action with a heart of hope. Feel gratitude, knowing that there is always hope for you—it's called God's grace.

WEDNESDAY: FIND THE FEARS, MOVE TO HOPE

"Don't lose hope. When it gets darkest, the stars come out."

—Anonymous

In *Freeing the Soul from Fear,* my wonderful mentor and teacher Robert Sardello suggests fear is always present in our world. Learning to work with hope in our hearts can help balance that fear and move us towards a hopeful heart.

Today is the day to find places in your life where fear makes you behave in ways you don't like, respect or admire. Being unconscious of fear allows it to grow, fester and prove itself right. The fear says, "See—I told you to be frightened. See what happened because you didn't follow my advice?"

Not all fear is bad, of course. Fear or feeling the need for caution can be a warning sign of *truly* dangerous situations and can help you make safe decisions. I don't step out in front of moving cars or walk down dark streets in dangerous areas or do things that I have a strong *knowing* not to do.

But many of our fears are imagined—beliefs that have sprung wrongly from our imaginations. (Remember my fear of the dark and the bogeyman as a little girl?) Today, review your fears and decide whether your fear is warning you of something real, or if it's imagined and falsely ruling your life. Where you recognize fear is driving your behavior, stop and see if it is the best motivator for you. Are you *really* in danger? And if not, reframe the situation from a hope-filled perspective.

I find sometimes I am frightened to say something to my husband, colleagues or friends—afraid they may react with anger or defensiveness or be upset. But in reality, nothing bad will happen if I say what I need to say, kindly, honestly and, mostly importantly, from my heart.

They may react angrily, but is that really a reason for the paralyzing fear in me? In fact, the friction may lead us to a resolution. If I don't address what is bothering me, that fear creates a barrier between us, and I behave in a resentful or angry manner. Consequently, the results are usually far worse than if I had chosen to operate with hope, speak from my heart and address what was bothering me.

When we are afraid to say something and bottle it up, one day it builds up so much we blurt it out as a fear-driven utterance or reaction, and then find ourselves in all sorts of strife. When we finally find the courage to face the same sort of situation with hope in our heart, the outcome is usually better.

Resentment can build up and up, and it influences how we interact with those around us, negatively in every way. We might *think* our resentment goes away, but it doesn't! Hope gives us the courage to say what we need to say.

For example, if I read an email and am concerned that there was an undercurrent of irritation in it, I can sit and fret and worry about it until it is a real issue for me. I become fearful that I have unknowingly done something wrong. Instead of this, I could call the person and from my heart say, "I read your email and I was wondering if I have done anything to upset you." Said in a soft, concerned voice *from the heart*, this usually gets a positive response and brings about resolution—if there was even anything to resolve. The critical part is to be honest with yourself and speak from your heart.

Pick one situation you are dealing with at the moment, and see if you can detect any fear surrounding it. If you do, find or breathe in hope, and see what inspiration comes with hope in your heart.

Most of our challenges and difficulties are in our imaginations. They are rarely real. Turn the light on (by that, I mean put hope into your heart) and see how the bogeymen have all gone away. A heart that is thinking correctly fears nothing.

THURSDAY: HOPEFUL EXPECTATIONS

"There is no medicine like hope, no incentive so great, and no tonic so powerful as expectation of something better tomorrow."

—Orison Marden

Today is the day of hopeful expectations. In other words, you are to go through this day expecting good things to happen. And for situations to work out perfectly, as God planned them, no matter what *you* think they should look like.

As you are driving or traveling to work, expect the traffic to flow easily or a seat to become available in public transport. If neither of these happen, be hope-full that there is a good reason for any difficulties and that this will become obvious at some point.

If you are full of anxiety about a meeting that you have been dreading, *stop!* And immediately become hope-full about it by giving the situation to God or "pre-living" it the way in which you would like to see it happen.

Imagine yourself living through the experience with all those hope/body sensations that you became aware of on Monday. Imagine having a positive outcome by feeling and operating in a hope-full and therefore courage-full way. Then, walk into the meeting with your new courage and hope "demeanor."

If someone who scares you is approaching and you stop breathing, seize up, clench your fists or sweat—know that fear has "gripped" you. Stop. Take a breath. Replace those fear sensations with hope-filled courage and from that new position, interact with this person. You might be stunned at the difference!

On your way home, be hopeful about how the evening will work out. Imagine things going well; your relationship being smooth and easy; your teenager succeeding in life despite the fact they appear to be totally uninterested in anything except aggravating you right now!

Feel what it is like to go through a day with hope, and hopeful expectations, instead of dread, worry, resignation and expecting the worst. Take notes and decide which feels better. Then make your choice of how to operate—from your heart's wisdom or your imagination or fabrication! Consciously choose hopeful expectations for the day.

Finally, make a list of all the things about which you would like to be hopeful. Really *feel* the hope in your heart as you write—it's not enough to just write it down. You have to consciously work to eliminate the fears, *feel* the hope and really believe in the possibilities in each situation. Breathe those possibilities into your heart.

You already know what it's like to wait full of dread and anxiety—wait for the worst to happen. So today and from now on, even if things don't work out the way you wanted them to, be full of positive, hopeful expectations, which will keep you in a good frame of mind while you are waiting. Maybe you will be in a better state to take what does happen and make something great out of it!

How you feel is up to you. Actively hold onto hope!

FRIDAY: TACKLE SOMETHING DIFFICULT WITH HOPE

"Most of the important things in the world have been
accomplished by people who have kept on trying when there
seemed to be no hope at all."

—Dale Carnegie

Think of a difficult situation in your life right now. Are you looking at
it through "glasses" made of fear or of hope? Do you have a sense that
all is, or will be, as it should be? Do you believe that even if something
unpleasant has happened as a result of someone else's free will run
amok, good can come of it?

Sometimes people who say "Everything happens for a reason" passively wait for the world to come to them. Believing things happen for
a reason does not mean we can sit back and do nothing. We *must* try to
be conscious of what is going on, fulfill our responsibilities and play our
part. If you don't know what to do, then say to yourself, "I don't know
what the best thing is to do, but I will have faith, do the right thing, be
loving, kind, compassionate and hopeful and see what unfolds."

Pick one of the most difficult life challenges you have right now.
Revise your thinking about it. No matter how hopeless it seems, work
with your will and use faith and hope in the person or the scenario to
instill yourself with the courage you need to do something (like work
on forgiveness or make plans to talk to the person or find a way to love
them fully or accept them).

If there really is nothing you can do, accept the situation and look
at it with hope-filled eyes and heart, knowing that spiritual wisdom is
at work and can change anything in an instant. Pray. You may do nothing different except change your thoughts or feelings, and everything
might change!

Hold the hope that you will be guided with inspiration to know
what to do, even if you don't know now. *Hope-fully* expect that insight
and clarity will come to you or the right people will appear or the right
situation will emerge. Your job is to be watchful and listen carefully for
that inspiration and to trust in the wisdom given to you.

Be conscious of which thoughts control you. If you are uncertain about what will happen, find hope and expect that good will come of it. When it does, it may not look "good" to you, but with the benefit of hindsight, you might see it turned out much better than you imagined. Remember, "hope springs eternal," as Alexander Pope wrote in 1733. It can keep us going, motivated and persistent when others give up.

The heart is an alchemical vessel in which hope is used to transmute everything difficult into something beneficial. Put all your problems in the heart, fill it with the philosopher's stone of hope, and see what emerges. (The philosopher's stone was the secret, magical ingredient used by alchemists to transmute base metals into gold.)

I never give up. Never. It drives my husband crazy! Hope gives me the energy to have persistence, resilience and optimism. And sometimes that persistence takes the form of patience—but not very often! I have to work on that one.

I do try, however, to make sure that what I am striving for is also what I believe to be God's will and not just me forging on until I have my own way. If I can't actually do anything, then I wait for inspiration to come for the next step. I know there is always a next step! I wait in hope, not in despair.

After all, what human knows what will happen in the future—this is the realm of alchemy and miracles!

SATURDAY: THE DIFFERENCE BETWEEN HOPE-ING AND HOPE-FUL

"The very least you can do in your life is figure out what you hope for. And the most you can do is live inside that hope. Not admire it from a distance but live right in it, under its roof."

—Barbara Kingsolver

There is a difference between wishing and hoping. Hope without faith is empty—it is simply wishing. Hope filled with faith is active. It spurs us on to *do something*.

We can wish all we like that things will change or be different, but wishing does nothing. It places all the power externally. We wish someone would come along and fix things so everything would be fine, but we do nothing to contribute! We don't take an active role.

I think many people say, "I'm hoping this situation is going to improve" without actually engaging in the whole process. It's just a word they use to describe the feeling of, "I have given up and am resigned to what will happen." (This is often accompanied by a sigh!) These people may still be living in fear but are just saying they are hopeful! They are really wishing things were different without being *willing* to be involved actively or consciously.

Our work is to maintain hope and faith. To live in hope, to step into hope, to put hope into our hearts for the alchemical process requires us to take action. We must hold onto faith, move, *do something* to see the world differently or change the way we react. We must be conscious of what sort of expectation we have—one of hope or one of dread?

When we really are full of hope, we are filled with light and actually *feel* lighter. We vibrate at a different rate and are actually different beings. Our hearts are different; we are conscious of the decision to operate from hope; we have *done something* to make that possible.

My husband, Ken, had an interesting experience with hope and our herbalist friend Mary. She assessed him and told me the things she had found, which I was to share with Ken. They were not necessarily easy things to hear, and I was being led by fear when I worried about his reaction. But when I did tell him, using hope and courage as my companions, he said *he* was filled with hope and light deep inside.

When Ken heard what Mary had found, he felt, at last, that someone had really identified what had been core issues for him. I believe Mary is inspired in her work, and Ken sensed her spiritual connection to God and to us, and he felt that what she spoke was truth for him. That gave him hope.

Ken has since been able to find that same sensation and fill himself with it rather than disappointment or another fear-based emotion. And he can choose a very different way of approaching the world now, especially when he catches himself having negative thoughts. Both of us still fall back into our old fear-based habits at times—but now we can recognize them, breathe and choose to become hopeful and expect good things to come.

Today, see if you can feel the difference between actively making your heart full of hope as opposed to just passively hope-ing or wishing for things to be transformed.

Hope comes with knowing, and choosing to remember, that the spiritual worlds will help when you need it. Go on—you can do it!

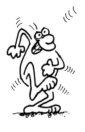

CHAPTER 4

A WEEK OF REVERENCE

"Always and in everything let there be reverence."

—Confucius

YOUR SEVEN MINUTES

What does "reverence" mean to you? Unfortunately, it's not a common conscious practice.

Reverence in its pure state is the ability to see God in everything and everyone and to hold that *spiritual* quality in awe. Do you remember reading of a reverential "fear" of God? From what I understand, this fear of God is actually a state of awe—having a reverential awe of the power and presence of God.

Think about the things or people you handle or treat with reverence. What or whom do you revere, honor or respect?

Do "things" keep coming up for you more than people or the spiritual worlds? Money? Possessions? Having more than others? Hopefully you think of awesome people for their qualities and not their money or fame! Do you think of nature, perhaps?

Where do you feel reverence in your body?

How do you show reverence? What are your behaviors, how do you use your body, and what is your voice tone like when you feel reverent?

AMANDA'S TAKE ON REVERENCE

"The moment I have realized God sitting in the temple of every human body, the moment I stand in reverence before every human being and see God in him—that moment I am free from bondage, everything that binds vanishes, and I am free."

—Swami Vivekananda

Have you ever seen the way the Nepalese, or some Indians and Buddhists, greet each other? They put their hands together as if in prayer, and bow their heads and say "Namaste," which has a variety of meanings around a similar theme: "The spirit in me salutes the spirit in you"; "I greet that place where you and I are one"; "The light within me sees and honors the light within you"; or simply—"I see God in you."

Would that not be a great way for us all to greet people? To be constantly reminded that in front of us stands an incredible, awesome being of light? Remember the pilot light that lives inside our hearts? Reverence ignites that pilot light of our spirit.

Reverence, like forgiveness, needs to be a way of living, and this greeting can be the trigger to remind us many times a day to treat everyone and everything with reverence.

You might feel silly walking up and saying Namaste in our culture, so when you meet someone, try to meet their spirit with your reverent smile or handshake. Try to make the greeting more meaningful than just, "Hi, how are you?"

At a class I attended recently, someone brought out an ancient treasure: a 3,000-year-old rose quartz Buddha. You should have seen how people handled that Buddha, and rightly so! It was worth millions of dollars but was priceless in terms of what it represented. It was irreplaceable. But it was just an *object*. I didn't see anyone else there handling another human in the same way!

How easily we can do that—have reverence for, and handle with awe and wonder, an external object whose value we measure by huge amounts of money or its uniqueness or irreplaceable nature. Yet we don't realize that in front of us every day stand one-of-a-kind beings of unimaginable beauty, spirit, value and worth.

How do we treat them? When did you last view a human with awe, wonder and reverence? We do it all the time with film stars and famous people—our culture has made them objects of awe and wonder, or of horror in some cases! But when did you last view someone with whom you live or work with awe and wonder?

We have forgotten about reverence in our culture, and it's time to bring it back to consciousness. Imagine how great it would be if we were all treated with, and treated others with, respect, awe, wonder and reverence.

I was touched by this section of a spectacular poem by Hafiz, one of the best-known Sufi poets from Persia, translated by Daniel Ladinsky:

MY BRILLIANT IMAGE

> *One day the sun admitted,*
> *I am just a shadow.*
>
> *I wish I could show you*
> *The Infinite Incandescence*
> *That has cast my brilliant image.*
>
> *I wish I could show you,*
> *When you are lonely or in darkness*
> *The Astonishing Light*
> *Of your own Being.*[1]

Imagine what the world would be like if we greeted each other daily in this way—if we could see the astonishing light of each being or at least imagine that it were there and greet it! Imagine if our politicians, corporations, corporate leaders and community leaders all remembered and were guided by the virtue of reverence.

ARROGANCE AND CRUELTY—ENEMIES OF REVERENCE

"Whoever undertakes to set himself up as a judge of truth and knowledge is shipwrecked by the laughter of the gods."

—Albert Einstein

One of the definitions of cruelty is heartlessness. If we act from our hearts, we behave with gentleness, kindness, respect and reverence. If we act from our fears or insecurities, we can be competitive, manipulative, controlling, political or just plain old mean!

It feels to me that the opposite of reverence is a blend of arrogance, pride and cruelty—a disregard for the life and light in others and therefore life itself—all arising from unconsciousness and detachment.

We don't even have to be arrogant to be cruel. We can be cruel unconsciously, or, more sadly, on purpose. Our tongues can be very cruel. Be careful and mindful of what you say to others and about others. Words can lift someone's spirit or crush it in a heartbeat. Are your words spoken in a tone of reverence?

Our actions can be cruel. Even our non-actions—such as not communicating with people. We may give someone the "cold shoulder," or have little "clubs" at work where we exclude people, or we may exclude people from our family circles. (Sometimes there is a real reason for not communicating. Instead, pray for those people from a distance.)

How do you treat others—always with kindness and respect or differently from that?

How much respect did Mother Teresa command throughout the world? And how did she treat *everyone*? With absolute reverence and love. Humility is the quality that goes hand in hand with reverence. Humility and reverence both acknowledge the source of our light. We need to reawaken our awareness of the qualities of humility and reverence—and weave them through *every* aspect of our lives.

Once we comprehend the *spiritual* nature of everyone and everything and accept that we are all connected, the whole and part of the whole, then we can no longer be cruel or arrogant. Instead, awe, wonder, humility and reverence will reign!

Michael Grinder, one of my mentors, says of nonverbal communication, "We are in love with the influence of power, when we should be in love with the power of influence." (His website is www.michael grinder.com and he offers great classes.) The same is true of the influence the spiritual worlds have on us—their power is awesome!

REVERENCE FOR THE WORLD, EARTH AND NATURE

"To believe that every tree, plant and insect can talk takes an open mind. Go by yourself into nature and sit quietly. Then pick up a rock and listen to your thoughts. After a while, put that rock down and pick up another rock. Your thoughts will change. These are the voices and the wisdom of the stone people. Many of the stone people are very old and very wise."[2]

—Don Coyhis

What *you* do affects all living creatures and our environment and ultimately affects what happens on Earth.

Every time we pass something into our air or water system, we are affecting *all* the life, animals and humans that rely on that system, and they feed into many other systems. It's a connected world.

Are you someone who consciously cares for the earth? Or do you throw things out your car window as you drive along, completely unaware and uncaring of the consequence?

Do you recycle if you have the chance? This is a way of showing reverence for the earth—instead of polluting her with all our landfill and toxins. Do you think carefully about cleaning products that you use? Seventh Generation is one company passionately committed to enhancing our lives and the environment.

Do you keep your car in good shape so you are not constantly spewing out products that harm people, and the earth?

Do you take the shopping cart out into the parking lot and leave it in the designated collection area? Or do you abandon it where it can roll and hit another car? Are you considerate when you drive? Or do you think the road is yours and everyone else is an idiot?

There are many small daily things that you can do if you *choose* to live and behave consciously, with reverence. *You* can make a big, positive difference to the whole.

Imagine a world where all companies treated the earth and people with reverence instead of revering the dollar, bottom line and profits. There would be a lot less corruption and many more fulfilled employees if companies focused on true serving and reverence as a mission statement and were not consumed by goals based on power and greed.

For instance, why would anyone treat a service-oriented person with less respect than they would a corporate executive? Without those service-oriented people doing their jobs, there might not be a corporate executive! And the people who are the first point of contact with customers are often the most important people in the company—they create the relationships that determine a sale, loyalty or great word-of-mouth advertising.

Large companies that care little for their employees or customers, and that consequently offer appalling service, have lost touch with what is really important for their businesses, i.e., building relationships through serving, revering, helping, supporting, taking care of their employees and customers and paying attention to how people *feel*.

I believe one of the reasons my husband is such a great leader is that he is naturally humble and has a real reverence for the people who work with him. He sees their potential and the possibilities in them and he tries to develop that.

His book, *The People Pill,* is in some ways a study of reverence in the corporate world. The companies he led had soaring profits under his leadership, and I am not just his biased wife! The actual figures are astounding—and he made them happen by engaging and developing people and treating them all with respect and reverence.

Reverence needs to be a part of everything we do. It's a daily gesture that can infuse every movement, and every moment, with the Divine.

HANDLING OBJECTS WITH REVERENCE

How do you put objects on a table? Do you chuck them down or throw them from a distance? It doesn't really matter what the item is, if you throw it down without any thought, you are creating a spiritual gesture of violence!

Think about it—when you see someone take your business card the way the Japanese do—with two hands and with great reverence—how does it make you feel? It makes me feel honored and respected.

If you take someone's business card but just shove it in your pocket, what have you just told that person nonverbally? It's the same with anything another person gives you—a document, manuscript, gift or food. Take it from them respectfully, treat it with care, and place it gently down. Try doing this for just one day—handle *everything* as if it were something very precious that had been given to you to keep safe. You will be amazed at how different you feel!

If you do this consciously, you will find that you can enter into a state of reverence—your cells will start to vibrate in harmony, in resonance with reverence, and this will have a dramatic impact on everything that you do while you remain in that state!

Throwing anything that isn't mean to be thrown carries that spiritual gesture of violence. If it's a football or a basketball, it's okay to throw it! But even then, *how* it is thrown is important—if the ball is thrown with the intent to hurt someone, it is neither respectful nor reverent to the person or even the principles of the game.

REVERENCE FOR FOOD AND OUR BODIES

Do you treat food with reverence? Do you see it for what it represents—your life-renewal force? Do you say grace and not only thank God, the cook and the farmers but also the food for the work it did in growing, and nature for providing you with this nourishment?

Many of us don't even *stop* to eat. We drive, work on the computer, do tasks, shop and catch up on our to-do list while we eat. Is that treating the food *or* our bodies with reverence? I love the way the French, as a culture, appreciate, savor and honor their food and the process of eating.

How we *prepare* food is significant! Even if you eat out all the time, pick your restaurants carefully so there is some care and love with the preparation of the nourishment you are providing for your body. Most of us see eating as some process that has to happen to stave off hunger, rather than a vital source of nourishment and life forces.

If we prepare food with love, care and reverence, those qualities go into it and feed us spiritually. If we just throw something together and shove it into our mouths, the gesture of reverence is absent—and much of the physical and spiritual nutritional value.

When you put food on the table, do you slam it down or place it with care and love as if it were a gift? If waiters did this and approached their jobs and guests with reverence, I bet they would earn a *lot* more in tips!

REVERENCE FOR YOUR SELF/YOUR SOUL

What are you doing to your mind? Do you fill it with negative, cruel and gruesome images? Do you watch violent movies or programs? Do you compare yourself with others constantly?

Do you beat yourself up with your negative internal dialogue? You can replace that dialogue by repeating a list of things that make you feel positive and light. Speak with reverence to *yourself*, not just to others.

If you forget to see God in yourself or other people and struggle to treat them with reverence, at least treat them, and yourself, with respect. And that means no screaming, shouting, hitting, cruelty, abuse or violence. It means having self-control, compassion and caring, and acting with kindness. Hopefully that will lead you to living in, and behaving with, reverence.

Do you educate yourself and learn new and interesting things? Do you have meaning in your life? Have you infused your work and your heart with a sense of purpose? Do you have friends who are uplifting and encouraging? Are you passionate about anything? Do you have hobbies that challenge and stimulate you?

What are you doing for your spirit? Do you take time to just sit quietly in natural surroundings and allow the peace of nature to restore you? Do you have faith in a higher power and take time to attune to it? Do you attend classes or do anything to learn or grow spiritually? Do you read uplifting books? Do you see your life as a service to others? These are some ways you can treat yourself with reverence.

Pretend when you speak with someone that the person is God. (I know a human is not God, but they have a God-like spirit inside them—they are part of God. So are you!) Would you dare to shout at or speak to God in a disparaging, belittling or nasty way? I doubt it.

Imagine that people walk around with a little sign on their forehead and it says, "God lives here." Treat them as if you had God standing in front of you—they will wonder what has happened to you! That's the power of love and reverence.

The gesture of reverence, both the physical and spiritual kind, is something we can weave into all our daily activities, and it will lead us to humility, joy and more true influence. It may help us develop a sense of purpose or meaning in life; it will certainly be rewarding and fulfilling and bring us satisfaction in more ways than we can imagine.

DAILY SCHEDULE

SUNDAY: REVERENCE FOR GOD, OUR ANGELS AND ALL THE SPIRITUAL BEINGS WHO HELP US

"Millions of spiritual creatures walk the earth unseen, both when we wake and when we sleep."

—John Milton

No matter what your spiritual belief system, we need to treat God (or your equivalent of God), angels, guides, nature spirits and all living things with awe, wonder and reverence.

Too often we forget about all the angels that help us out—on earth and from "above." I believe we have guardian angels and that there are many "angels" in human guise who help us through our lives. They come in all shapes and sizes and appear magically at the times we need them, and it is only afterwards that we realize we were "touched by an angel." Awesome!

This is the realm of miracles and things way beyond our understanding, so just be grateful that we are living in a world where miracles can and do happen all the time. Be very reverent towards this whole amazing, awe-inspiring spiritual world of which we are members!

Look around you today and try to feel God in all you do; be aware of all the beings that are with us as well, like loved ones who have passed and angels who want to help us. They *are* there. We just don't know how to look, sense, feel and listen for them. It's easy-ish! Be quiet, look with your heart and listen.

At the wake after Mum's funeral, I was standing on the balcony talking with one of her oldest and dearest friends, my surrogate mum, Billee, when a turquoise butterfly flew right by me—two stories up. I saw it and instantly knew it was Mum! It was the strangest thing. I just *knew* it. Turquoise was one of her favorite colors.

Several days later when I was really missing her, I was with some friends on their farm. For three hours I was surrounded by all manner of turquoise bugs—butterflies, dragonflies and others I could not even recognize. Since then, Mum has sent me many butterflies—they appear on billboards, in airports, in magazines and in cards. It's my inner knowing that makes it true for me.

I have told this story many times now, and almost everyone has a similar one. Those who have crossed the threshold are always with us—we just need to wake up and recognize their presence! How could you not be filled with wonder and reverence at the amazing ways they can connect with us?

Thank God for all He has done for you, for all the help He has sent you, the blessings, gifts and grace He has bestowed on you, and for His ongoing forgiveness. We have a lot to revere! Treat Him with respect; do not ignore Him; listen carefully for what He has to say to us; take time with Him every day; and sit in awe, wonder and gratitude for everything we have been given.

Listen for His will and align yours with His. It works out better in the end. Much better! I love what C.S. Lewis wrote: "There are two kinds of people: those who say to God, 'Thy will be done' and those to whom God says, 'All right, then, have it your way!'" The price is much greater if we do it our way.

MONDAY: REVERENCE FOR LIFE

> "By having a reverence for life, we enter into a spiritual relation with the world. By practicing reverence for life, we become good, deep and alive."
>
> —Albert Schweitzer

Life is a precious gift that we largely ignore until it is about to be taken away or changed dramatically. A life-threatening illness or event usually transforms a person's perspective. Have you met anyone who has survived cancer, fought off another catastrophic illness or had a near-death experience? Almost everyone will tell you that they have a newfound reverence for life, and for everyone and everything in their world; they now enjoy every moment.

Why do most of us wait for a crisis to start appreciating what we have? Because most of us are asleep and take our life forces for granted! We are unconscious of the beauty, joy and wonder of being alive. We are living life at half-mast.

Imagine you were told you had a month to live. That's all. One month. *How* would you live in that last month—not what would you do, but *HOW would you live*? This may be the most important question in this whole book. It is at critical times like this that many people discover their true spiritual nature. Many people who have never prayed before or believed in prayer or a God or anything spiritual start to pray with fervor at times of crisis. They develop faith, which Gandhi says "is nothing but a living, wide-awake consciousness of God within."

I hope you would suddenly start treating life with great reverence and that you would recognize how precious it is. That you would see everything in your life as a gift—your family, friends, colleagues, difficulties, challenges, even your enemies would look pretty good at that time!

I hope you would look longingly at nature's magnificence, and the tiniest things would bring joy, wonder and awe; that you would suddenly see the bigger picture and not be caught in petty squabbles; that you would not waste time watching mindless television instead of communicating with your family and friends; that you would explore and share your feelings; and that you would be honest and truthful.

Art Buchwald, the famous American journalist, was told in 2006 that he was going to die. His kidneys had failed in June, and he was given three weeks to live and went into a hospice. He was cared for and nurtured, spent time with his family and friends, and *relished* every moment of life. As he told the story later, he was full of joy and had a great time, and developed a deep sense of reverence for life.

Five months later, he had to check out of the home because his kidneys were now functioning. Joy, reverence, gratitude and relishing every moment of his life restored his life! He died in January 2007 after he had written another book called *Too Soon to Say Goodbye!* published by Random House.

Today is the day to look at how you respect and revere your life. Start being conscious of every wonderful moment you are given—whether it is disguised as a challenge or is an obvious blessing. Become full of reverence for it and for *everything* that happens and for all those who are in your life. Be glad, joyful, grateful and kind, and relish every little thing that happens—all the pain, challenges, difficulties and the fun. Treat your life as the precious and wonderful gift it is.

A good friend sent me an email that talked about how God is in charge of the "knots and strings" in our lives. They are like the knots under a lovingly handwoven rug. When it is finished and you turn the rug over, it feels smooth and has a magnificent pattern. If we only looked at the knotted side, we would only see chaos. Knowing that God is weaving a beautiful pattern is awesome!

TUESDAY: REVERENCE FOR NATURE

"Gratitude bestows reverence, allowing us to encounter everyday epiphanies, those transcendent moments of awe that change forever how we experience life and the world."

—John Milton

It's almost impossible to talk about reverence without mentioning awe and wonder.

PROJECT 1: FEEL AWE, WONDER AND REVERENCE FOR NATURE

Go out today and find some aspect of nature to bring those feelings to you. Plan a weekend trip to immerse yourself in it. If that is impossible, find some spectacular photos and lose yourself in them. Put those photos up on walls around you so you can be aware of, and *feel,* the majesty of nature with awe, wonder and reverence.

On a trip to Nashville's Opryland to speak, I was in one of many long corridors on the way to my room. For those of you who have not been to this famous, amazing hotel and conference center in Nashville, it is enormous! It covers five acres and you have to walk miles (it seems) to reach the meeting rooms, and it is very easy to find yourself lost in all those corridors.

I was irritated and lost, and a family emerged from another corridor. They were obviously lost as well. The father was angrily pushing a luggage cart that was overloaded and the mother was busy looking at a map trying to work out where they were. They had two small children aged about four and six who were having the best time! They were dancing and jumping with excitement even though they were in a windowless corridor!

This to me was a blinding-flash-of-the-obvious moment. Suddenly I saw awe and wonder contrasted directly against how we have come to live our lives as adults. The adults were frustrated, angry and upset. The children were finding the joy in the situation—they were full of awe, wonder and laughter, and made the experience fun by playing.

As adults, we are so engrossed with being on a mission (like finding the room), *doing* stuff and *having* stuff that we forget to look around and feel awe and wonder for where we are. It's easy to be filled with awe when we look at a magnificent view, as I am doing now, experiencing the amazing beauty of nature and the incredible silence of our little farmhouse in Vermont.

Consider the ocean and its unfathomable power, or look at the night sky in all its vastness. Think about the Grand Canyon, or being in ancient forests or rain forests, or being beside rivers and isolated streams, or watching ants and what they can do. Any of this can fill us with awe, wonder and reverence and feed our souls. There is something in the silence, vastness and wisdom of nature that makes us become conscious of reverence.

Go out today and become conscious of the amazing power of the natural world surrounding you.

PROJECT 2: PRACTICE EVERYDAY REVERENCE

Find a way to look at everyday-life situations with awe and wonder—like those children in the halls of Opryland did. We all did that as children, so we all have the capacity to do it—just as we have the innate capacity for joy. It sits patiently inside us waiting for the day, like today, when we will awaken to it.

No matter what happens today—find a reason to be in awe and wonder.

Look at your colleagues and family with a sense of awe for the incredible spiritual beings they are. They may be covered with a pretty ordinary personality, but they are really "astonishing beings of light"!

Be amazed at the technology of your car—that it can take you places and you never need to think about it—unless it doesn't work!

Find yourself in awe of how the universe or God or Source arranges everything so perfectly—no matter how messy it looks to us!

I am always fascinated and in awe of people who can create machinery or make art or carve wood into glorious shapes. I'm also fascinated and awed by people who manage very difficult lives and still smile, or by people with severe handicaps who are so grateful for what they have.

I stand in awe of doctors and healers who can work magic, and on and on. I look at everyone with curiosity, fascination and wonder—how can they do what they do?

Everyone—no matter who they are or what they do—has something amazing to give to life—and to us. We just need to be curious and look beyond ourselves to see it.

I see the world as an alive, swirling mass of awesome, amazing, wonderful, mysterious stuff just waiting for me to learn about it, and it's very exciting!

Remember the children in that corridor—part of your mission today is to experience everything with a sense of awe and wonder. You will be surprised at how much gratitude and joy you feel at the end of the day.

WEDNESDAY: REVERENCE FOR OTHERS

"Everybody can be great because anybody can serve. You don't have to have a college degree to serve. You need only a heart full of grace."

—Martin Luther King, Jr.

Namaste. That is your meditation for today. Silently greet every person you meet and every animal and plant you encounter with this word. In your imagination, feel yourself performing the gesture that goes with it, as you bow with reverence to the life force, to the "*I AM*" in front of you.

It's not weird to be greeting all life forms in this way. Plants are precious—they give us oxygen, herbs, food and a gazillion other things. They have their own life force—some see that life force as a spiritual being. Are you not amazed at how a seed can fall on the ground and, despite all the obstacles it has to overcome, emerge as a gorgeous flower or some nutrition-filled substance for you or animals to eat? Whether you see a bunch of flowers or a single bloom, try to grasp the amazing powers that went into creating them.

Animals are equally complex. Think of how they live, and survive, despite what humankind is doing to them and their environment.

When you see a squirrel or birds downtown, imagine what they have had to do to adapt to concrete jungles, not to mention how they can now eat junk food!

Remember, God is in every person you see. The beggar on the street, the janitor, the cab driver, your colleagues, the person who collects your trash, the corporate executive, the gardener, the cleaning person, the council worker, bus drivers, salespeople, cash register clerks—everyone! And most importantly, God is in your family.

Today is a special day for your family! You are going to treat them all as the precious spiritual teachers they are. They give us more opportunities to grow and develop than anyone else ever could.

You may not be the easiest person on the planet to live with in truth! Be in awe and wonder that they chose you! Be filled with reverence for them and gratitude that they are with you, and willing to *stick with you.* If they choose not to stick with you, be full of reverence anyway, because their departure may turn out to be the best thing that ever happened to you—no matter how bleak it looks at the moment.

Look for what is inside other people's hearts—this is their true nature and who they *really* are. *Everyone* is an astonishing being of light inside his or her heart. Feel blessed to have these people as part of your life. The blessing may not be obvious at this moment, but live in joyful, hopeful expectation that you will one day soon see that blessing.

You will be filled with awe and wonder at the magic that happens when you live with, and actively feel and show, reverence and respect for all.

THURSDAY: REVERENCE FOR YOUR SOUL AND SPIRIT

> "There is a Beautiful Creature
> Living in a hole you have dug."[3]
>
> —Hafiz

This is your day! The day for you to discover for yourself what a spectacular and awesome being you are. Try not to let judgments and critical thoughts come pouring in as you read that last line—they are the "hole" we have dug for ourselves. The more negative self-talk we have running in continuous loops through our minds, the deeper the hole.

Look at yourself through your heart today—*feel* who you really are. When we ask someone, "Who are you?" they mostly reply with what they do. "My name is Amanda and I am a motivational speaker"—or a banker, a manager, a nurse or mechanic, and so on.

That's not who we are! We are souls and spirits constantly creating our lives, merging with and connecting to God and others. It's the layers of personality and ego that block our vision of who we really are.

People like the Dalai Lama can see through all that ego and personality stuff because they know who we are in our hearts, and they wear the glasses of compassion, which, like X-ray vision, cut through.

Pretend for today that you are the loving parent of you—the child! That this is the day God is going to help you see your real self—remember, He *is* your loving parent! When you see yourself as He does you will automatically treat yourself with reverence. There is something for your soul to do in this world—some special purpose that only you can do.

You may be a little flawed—we all are—but that is because you are human. You are not a loser, victim, failure, hopeless, difficult, troubled or any other label you, or someone else, has attached to you.

We are responsible, special spiritual beings; we need to acknowledge our limitless nature and capacity, and be actively doing what we were meant to be doing on this journey. We treat our purpose and spiritual work with reverential awe. We do what we must do to discover what that purpose and work is, learn about it, and do it the best we can.

So today find out who you really are and what your spiritual purpose is and begin to fulfill it! Have a chat with God and ask Him who you are and what His will is for you.

Watch only uplifting TV programs; read spiritual books; listen to or attend a spiritual class; spend time on your own; reflect on your limitless nature; and see yourself as important, special and valuable. Surround yourself with beauty—flowers or photos or scenery; have *wonder*-ful aromatherapy oils burning so your sense of smell is pampered. (Pure aromatherapy oils and their scents can lift the spirits tremendously.) Hang out with people and friends you love, and go away for relaxing weekends or days.

These may not sound like ways to treat yourself with reverence, but they are! When you do activities that help you relax and reconnect with yourself, God, your family and friends, you are doing something spiritual and acknowledging your true nature, coming into harmony with it.

FRIDAY: REVERENCE FOR YOUR BODY

"He who loses his reverence for any part of his life will lose his reverence for all of his life."

—Albert Schweitzer

This is a *big* day! Hopefully it is the start of a new way of treating your body—the temple that houses your spirit.

I don't want to hear any laughter about your body being a ruined or crumbling temple! If, however, it is not a temple in great shape, today is the day to change that.

Without your body, you have no life on earth. It really *is* a temple and it does house your soul and spirit so it's pretty important in the big scheme of things. If it functions well and is healthy, then you have more energy to do your spiritual work. There may seem to be a lot to do here—but just choose aspects that resonate with you and it won't seem so daunting.

First, acknowledge and thank your body for keeping you going as well as it has to date, and humbly apologize for the stresses to which you have exposed it. And then promise to take better care of it, starting today.

The body needs to be in harmony with the world and nature's rhythms. We need about seven hours of sleep most nights. We need to balance sedentary activity with exercise, which is critical for a healthy body. We need rhythmic patterns of eating healthy foods and drinking plenty of pure water. We need sunlight on our skin. We need to balance stress and stimulation with relaxation.

How much rhythm and balance do you have in your life?

Examine your life and identify your patterns today—and then pick one that is not so nourishing for your body and change it.

Perhaps you can set a rhythm of going to sleep, or at least being in bed, by 10 p.m. and waking up at 6 a.m. This gives you a great length of time to sleep—and it may seem artificial, but try it before you scoff! Many people are sleep-deprived these days, yet good sleep is one of the most essential requirements for treating your body with reverence. It revives, restores and renews every cell and life process.

Choose to regularly exercise. (After checking with a medical professional, of course.) At the very least, buy a pedometer and make sure you walk the ideal number of steps for you a day—it's not as bad as it sounds! (If you are exercising *too* much, do less!)

Hugs and massage are not just relaxing—they are critical. The skin is the largest organ in the body and it performs many important functions such as detoxing and it needs a good scrubbing periodically! Humans need touch—babies born prematurely who are massaged and touched frequently are out of their neonatal units faster than those who are not touched and they have fewer developmental problems. That's how *life-giving* touch is to humans. Book a massage for *yourself* today.

Find ways to bust stress. Stop any illegal drug use and/or stop smoking. Balance your alcohol intake—"moderation in everything" might be a cliché, but there is truth in it.

Create an "unwind" ritual for your journey home each night. Keep a notebook in the glove box, and before you start the car, write down your to-do list for the next day. Then put the notebook back, drive home and be present when you arrive instead of worrying about work. Or hang your troubles on a "trouble tree" outside your front door so that you come home to your family free of those burdens. If necessary, you can collect them again the next morning when you leave home!

Meditate at the same time every day. Pick a time that works for you and then just do it. For five to ten minutes, sit and focus on your breathing, a color, silence or the sound *om*. Do this several times a day for shorter periods if you are really under pressure. Do *some*thing that de-stresses you every day.

Doing these things will be treating your "temple" with reverence and the respect it deserves. Give your body a chance to help you like it wants to. At the very least, stop doing things that harm your body!

SATURDAY: **REVERENCE FOR YOUR FOOD**

Grace is not just a prayer we mindlessly say over our meal; it's a way of transmuting our food into physical and spiritual nourishment.

Decide that from today on, you will only use the best-quality fuel to power your temple/body. No more sodas with high-fructose corn syrup, ever! No more diet drinks. No trans fats. Read all the labels on your food. Minimize the amount of processed and prepackaged foods you buy. Make more of your own meals and prepare them with love and gratitude. At least for today!

Buy as much organic food—or at least hormone- and antibiotic-free food—as you can afford to (especially potatoes and other root vegetables, as ground vegetables absorb more pesticides and chemicals). Eat chickens and eggs that are truly free-range—the rest can be loaded with hormones and may affect our body systems *and* the environment.

Buy the book *Nourishing Traditions* by Sally Fallon (or find it at your library) and decide to cook meals at home as much as possible from now on. Stop eating out every night, or having takeout, or eating prepackaged foods. The nutritional value of most processed foods is minimal. And they are generally not prepared and cooked with love and care.

Have as much vegetable variety as you can and use what is in season. Try to eat local products as much as possible, as they are fresher and may still have some of their nutritional substances available to you. Make the effort to find food that has been allowed to mature on the vine, tree or plant. If you can't buy food that is fresh from the vine, often manufacturers pick organic food fresh and freeze it right in the field.

Having chosen your food with great consciousness and prepared it with love, care and thought, say grace over everything you eat or drink and thank God for it. Thank the plants and animals that contributed to this meal, and ask God to bless it and make it nutritious and healthy for your body in all ways.

Then eat it slowly and thoughtfully, with appreciation and reverence. And chew each mouthful 30 times! YES, you can do it!

Doing *everything* with reverence is a great sign that God is in everything you do.

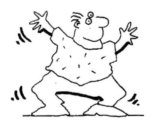

CHAPTER 5

A WEEK OF GENEROSITY, GIVING AND RECEIVING

"We make a living by what we get, but we make a life by what we give."

—Winston Churchill

YOUR SEVEN MINUTES

Are you a giving person? Do you have a generous heart and spirit? Is it easy for you to give freely—not just things but of yourself?

Who is the most generous person you know—not just, or only, financially?

How well can you receive and accept love, gifts or blessings? Is it easy for you? If someone compliments you, how do you respond? Do you believe you deserve good things?

Some people do nothing but receive, and rarely give! These people can have an "entitlement" mentality—they believe that they deserve to be given everything. Do you know anyone like that? Do you consider them generous of spirit?

AMANDA'S TAKE ON GENEROSITY, GIVING & RECEIVING

"The wise man does not lay up his own treasures. The more he gives to others, the more he has for his own."

—Lao-tzu

MAKE GENEROSITY A WAY OF LIVING

When people see or hear the word *generosity,* they first think of it in relation to money. Now is the time to think beyond that.

Money has its place, but more important is the deeper *quality* of generosity and making it a way of life for us. What are we willing to give? What is our motivation when we do give? In what spirit are we giving?

Someone with a generous spirit is continuously giving in many senses and ways; it is natural for them. They share their heart, time, love, thoughts, life, joy, gifts, possessions *and* their money! Some of the most generous people I know have very little money. But they are very rich!

Can you imagine living with a spirit of generosity in all aspects of your life? What would you be doing differently from what you do now?

Be generous in all ways. Be generous with your thinking; give people the benefit of the doubt and avoid judging. Give your time—it is the most precious gift one can receive. Share your knowledge and try to help everyone succeed. Be thoughtful.

If you see that a couple needs some time alone, do you offer to look after their children overnight? Or if you know someone needs help but cannot afford it, you give them the money to pay for it? My friend Mary does all this in the spirit of helping others—she is truly generous in all ways. And it just comes naturally to her. The more we practice this, the more naturally it will flow *from* us and *for* us!

IT'S ALL ABOUT THE FLOW OF LOVE

We live in a world held together with love—we just need to trust it is there, receive it and share it.

Generosity and gratitude go hand in hand. When we are grateful for love, our life and all that we receive, we understand how important it is to *share* the gifts in order to keep the flow of love going. That's what generosity is about—the flow of love in our world. *Anything given with a loving spirit is a wonderful gift.*

It doesn't matter what form the generosity flows in—it may be knowledge; it may be time; it may be money; or kindness or thoughtfulness, or any number of "things." What is important is that there is a loving intention which keeps love flowing out of you.

That love comes to us from God, not to hoard, keep and use selfishly. It is there to help us, so we can prosper and grow, but it's also there to pass on and help others prosper and grow. When we are generous, it expands our spirits, it brings us light and joy, it lights up others' lives, and it always has a win-win outcome!

THE IMPORTANCE OF RECEIVING

Almost as important as giving is the ability to receive. Without the receiving, there can be no flow. What is given hits a brick wall, slides down, and sits like a blob on the ground!

We need to be able to receive God's love and blessings, and love from others. Often we are given blessings and healings that we don't accept or receive, and they "sit" in our auras, waiting for us! All we have to do is say thank you and allow them in.

Babies and toddlers are giant sponges of receiving. They love to be loved. And in turn, they give so much joy and love back. They know about flow!

Modern lifestyles and cultures often leave children feeling unlovable, fearful, unworthy and unhappy. They have great trouble as adults receiving love, acknowledgment or recognition and allowing it to enter their hearts because they were so hurt or wounded.

It's a worthwhile exercise to examine and, if necessary, improve our ability to receive love; to know we are worthy of love and love-able! No matter what we have or have not done, God loves us and always will. Sometimes I think we love dogs and other animals because we can actually receive love from them—it's humans that make us wary!

If you don't feel worthy of love, look inside and see what you are saying to yourself that causes you to feel this way. If there are behaviors that you need to change to feel better about yourself, make the commitment and a plan. Just taking time to reflect on whether we feel worthy to receive love, help or blessings is something the vast majority of people never do. Become conscious of anything holding you back from freely giving *and receiving*.

I bet a lot of people really love you—even if they are not your parent! If you open your eyes and open your heart at the same time, you may be surprised at just how lovable you really are! Quirky maybe—but definitely lovable!

IT'S MY PIE AND I'LL KEEP IT IF I WANT TO!

Sharing it makes the pie bigger!

Generosity has an expansive quality about it. When we are generous, our spirit goes out to others, our love envelops others—we are described as "big hearted" or having a "big spirit." So the opposite would be a shrinking away of our being and spirit from others and from love. We shrivel up and become wizened, mean old critters! And perhaps it establishes the mind-sets for us to shrink away from our responsibilities as well.

The opposite of generosity is a state of shrinking away plus or minus selfishness, stinginess, isolation and fear.

Which makes me wonder about selfishness. What is selfishness really? We all are selfish in some way, and in certain areas of our lives— we think about ourselves, and we need to at times for growth and development—this *wise* selfishness is necessary. But "foolish" selfishness (as the Dalai Lama calls it), when we think *only* of ourselves and ignore the impact we inevitably have on others, can be harmful.

If we think only of what we want, have and need, and ignore the fact that we are all connected, part of the whole and have the whole within us, we forget that we *always* affect others! We are all part of a giant community—our souls are connected at very deep levels. When we cut off that connection, we shrink away and become "foolish" selfish. It harms us *and* others.

I wonder if the opposite of generosity is disconnection from the whole, which leads to fear (which perhaps led to the disconnection in the first place?)—so we then lose our perspective that everything we do affects everyone else at some level.

Generous, giving people trust, and they think of the effect they can have on others. They are not focused on hoarding and protecting what they have—or fearful of losing what they *think* they have. They recognize the whole and their role in the whole. Being stingy, selfish and mean-spirited stunts us and disconnects us from God's love and light.

Mean-spirited people almost visibly shrink and darken—physically and spiritually! Their mouths are tight, their brows are furrowed, they hold tightly onto things, they are miserable, and they hunch over and grumble a lot—think of Dr. Seuss's Grinch! They are very fearful of losing *all* they have if they give *any* of it away.

This type of person is also rarely grateful. They almost always feel as if they deserve more; that someone received more than they did. They are into comparisons: "I want what the Joneses have" or "Why can't I have that?" They want, and believe they deserve, all that *you* have, and feel no desire to return the generosity. (Maybe it's because they cannot receive love easily and they think love might come if they have more stuff!)

Disconnected, stingy, mean-spirited people unknowingly stop the flow of love. They receive and *keep,* out of fear! They do this rather than receive and *give,* not trusting that giving is what keeps love flowing to them and to others! Sometimes this type of behavior is called a poverty mentality: if you have some of the pie, there will be less for me. That is so *not* the way the cosmos works! We always make the pie bigger when we share with, give to and help others. It really is a matter of trusting rather than fearing.

If you help others at work by giving them your time, the benefit of your knowledge, and the wisdom you have gained from your experience, it will usually improve your position—not that you do it for that reason or with the expectation of receiving anything in return. This is especially effective if someone asks you for help first. Remember, it's sometimes good to wait till someone asks for help. Once asked, you can choose to give freely, no strings attached. (Check every so often that what you are sharing is actually what they want, and need!)

As a consequence, people will respect you and see you as an expert. Other people will also notice—perhaps your boss, and the next thing you know, you may be promoted! So instead of keeping all your wisdom to yourself, thinking, "If I keep this to myself, I am in a better position," share, expand, grow, focus on giving to others, and watch your life become full of light.

Having a generous spirit also means you have the right motivation— to give without *any* expectation of a return. You give because you want to give. Do it *especially* if you don't want to help or give.

Giving love is always appropriate, and often most effective, when we don't feel like doing it yet still make the choice to do it. People don't even need to know you are giving. It's enough that *you* know you are doing the right thing and sharing love.

BE GENEROUS WITH EVERYONE

"Thousands of candles can be lit from a single candle, and the life of the candle will not be shortened. Happiness never decreases by being shared."

—Buddha

Some of us are generous with our own families and no one else, and some of us are generous with others and not with our families. Review your life and see if you give your family enough of you—your time, energy, love and care. Feeding them and clothing them is good, but it is not generous. Being generous and giving them *you* is how to show you really love them and how you model the flow of love.

Are you bright, happy, entertaining and witty in public with strangers around you, and miserable and nasty at home? If so, you might want to consider your spirit of giving and think about where it is hiding!

True generosity has a purity in it that comes from having no motivation other than to *give* love, to *be* love, and to *share* love with others. Bring light to their lives—light their candles—and make sure the flow continues.

DAILY SCHEDULE

SUNDAY: BE GENEROUS WITH YOUR SPIRIT

"Every man must decide whether he will walk in the light of creative altruism or in the darkness of destructive selfishness."

—Martin Luther King, Jr.

Altruism is the quality of unselfish concern for the welfare of others. Today is your day to be creative and see how you can joyfully be generous and allow your spirit to shine its incredible glow on others.

It would be wonderful if we could realize how bright our light is and help others recognize their own astonishing light! We are all designed to be the candle that lights a thousand others. It's our choice whether to do it or not.

Will you do that today? Go out and consciously "light as many candles" as you can. Feel light and be light-filled, feel great and joyful, then spread that joy. Laugh, be happy, have fun and create joyful moments for you and for others.

If you are not feeling joyful, remember Psalm 118:24, which says, "This is the day the Lord hath made, we will rejoice and be glad in it." Notice that it's a conscious decision—we *will* rejoice and be glad!

Create ways to feel good, be joyful and give joy. Skip, dance, play, laugh, sing, admire nature, admire others and tell others they are wonderful and that you love them. In French, it's called *joie de vivre*—the joy of living! Use *your* joy today to bring joy and color to those around you.

Perhaps today you will just sit quietly, hold someone's hand and be with them. Whatever they need, generously give it to them.

Whatever it takes—commit yourself today to lighting up others and the world with your astonishing generous spirit.

MONDAY: BE GENEROUS WITH YOUR TIME

Just because you can't do everything, you should still do *everything you can.*

Time is one of the most precious commodities we have. Love is the *most* precious, and we should love enough to give our time. This is an investment with an abundant return. After we have passed, it will live on in those in whom we have invested and in whom they love and so on.

Today is the day for reflection on the time you give to others, especially your children, partners and parents.

Is it really *so* important that you have a fancy expensive car and large television in every room if it means you have to work so hard that you rarely see your children while they're awake? If you have a hobby or sport that takes you away from your family in the only spare time you have, you need to find a balance between giving to yourself and giving to those who love you.

Parents who are elderly and living alone need special attention. We think they are just fine and we call infrequently—and yes, they have their own lives, but many are older and more fragile than we realize. They may need more loving care than we currently give them.

One of the hardest things I had to deal with after Mum died was my regret over the *quality* of the time I gave her when I was with her. I spoke to her every day, visited her in Australia once or twice a year, and tried to do things with her that she liked to do. But I would also fix up everything that *I thought* needed to be fixed up and bought and sorted out.

I was very busy *doing* stuff for my mum but I didn't spend nearly enough time just *being* with her. It might have been just sitting and saying nothing sometimes, or having a drink with her and chatting, or telling her about what I was thinking and feeling and what was going on in my life. It might have been just listening to her talk about whatever she wanted.

I know in my heart that my mum wanted this more than anything, but I could not see it with my eyes because I had all these *things* to *do* for her. *Wrong!* Don't make the same mistake I made. Balance the *stuff* you have to *do* around your loved ones with just *being* with them and loving them—*and letting them love you.*

Even if you can't be with your parents physically, call them at least once a week and *do nothing else* while you are on the phone. Hear them with your heart and they will feel loved. This may be your last conversation with them so always make it a good one.

People debate the merits of quality versus quantity when it comes to spending time with people, but I reckon we need both. We need to give *lots* of good quality time. Try to spend more time with your parents. Even if you only have five minutes, it's still a wonderful gift when you are there in body, heart, mind and spirit.

We so often feel aggravated about the time we have to spend with people when we are rushed or busy, and it usually shows. If this is the way you find yourself, it's better you spend less time with them but have the right spirit. To be really present while we are with someone means we have to give them our *undivided* attention and listen. Stop the judging and self-talk that says, "I don't have time for this" or "Hurry up, will you?" or even, "Here we go again, the same old story."

Most of our parents made a lot of sacrifices for us. It's a small price to pay to return some of the love they gave us in the past. It's all about flow, remember?

Make time today to be fully present with the most important people in your life, and then make some time for yourself. See if you can establish a rhythm where you can continue to be there for them, and yourself, in some way. You will see great joy in the eyes of the people for whom you do this.

TUESDAY: **GIVE FROM YOUR HEART**

"Let no one ever come to you without leaving better and happier. Be the living expression of God's kindness: kindness in your face, kindness in your eyes, kindness in your smile."

—Mother Teresa

Giving from the heart, for me, means that we are open and honest, and that we gently share how we *feel* (rather than just spewing out our emotions). We give or share for the right reasons; we are kind; we have compassion; we care; we do everything with love.

It's through the heart that we connect with God, so to give from your heart is to give to others as God gives to you—always with love, always freely and always with grace, even when you don't "deserve" it.

Gifts that come from the heart are the gifts that money can't buy. This could be letters to your parents, partner or children that tell them what they mean to you, how special they are, what you love about them, and much more. Mum used to write me these letters and of course, I always cried with joy when I read them.

I had those letters all carefully stored when I moved to the U.S., but one of my greatest regrets in life is that a storage shed I rented was flooded and the storage company did not let me know. (Be wary of companies that are not members of an official association!) Without my knowledge, that company threw away many of my material possessions, including the most treasured ones, those letters from my mum. (I am still working on forgiveness!) But at least I have the memory of those letters, if not the actual papers.

After she passed, I was cleaning Mama's apartment and I found the letters I had sent to her. She had kept them together in a special place in her apartment. You never know how much a gift of the heart like that will mean to another person. If you have not written a similar letter to someone you love, today is the day! You might feel like you want to write five of them. Wonderful!

A gift of the heart can be sending loving thoughts to a person or holding them in your heart, or giving them something you have created lovingly that they might treasure or enjoy. It might be as simple as giving your attention. (Just noticing someone and saying good morning may be transformational for that person.) Try a kind word, a small compliment or a big compliment!

Smile at someone with kind eyes. Send a supportive glance to someone who is being yelled at. Write a friend a letter. Send an email to say "I am thinking of you." Send flowers for no reason. Jot down a note that says how much you value the effort someone put in for you, or write a note that tells your child how proud you are of them and how much you love them.

There are a million ways you can be the "living expression of God's kindness." Chances exist every day for you to do that.

Today is the beginning of a new life of giving from your heart—consciously and willingly!

WEDNESDAY: GIVE TO YOURSELF AND RECEIVE IT

Don't give up; just give!

Many people are generous with others and really mean-spirited to themselves. They rarely give themselves any love, credit, care, grace, any *thing* or any *time*—for resting, recuperation, joy, spiritual renewal, learning, fun, balance, being alone, health or exercise.

If we live like this, we burn out and don't have the energy or spirit to be generous because it's all we can do to make it from day to day. And often we become martyrs—a state that definitely doesn't have a spirit of generosity!

We can't continuously give to others without *allowing* something to flow back in—the most renewing source is God's love! Remember, it is a *flow*. If you are not surrounded with humans who give to you and balance the flow, you can always go directly to God, who is pouring grace and blessings out to you continuously. Ask for and *receive* those blessings. He even tells us to "ask and ye shall receive"—our job is to allow His love into our hearts.

For the full flow, there has to be generous giving and active receiving. Are you giving *yourself* enough gifts to keep you in that flowing stream?

By "gifts," I mean the gift of time to yourself to do something you love to do: to exercise; to stop and have a quiet moment somewhere; to go somewhere special to celebrate; to play a sport; to hang out with friends you have not seen for ages; to have a bath; or to read a book.

And doing things *for* yourself doesn't mean you have to do things *by* yourself!

Find ways to make activities do double duty—for example, housework. Instead of perceiving it as an onerous chore, choose to perceive it as being fun and rewarding! If you could teach your whole family that this shared activity is rewarding and fun, there might be several of you sharing the housework and then everyone wins.

Listen today for any words you say to yourself that are not full of grace and kindness. Who are you to say you don't deserve grace when God has decided you do?

Remember, you will never be perfect—no one will. All you can do is be the best you can be each day. And do your best again the next day. This is the gift of patience.

The gift of self-love and self-acceptance is a lifetime journey for most of us. (Self-loathing is easy!)

I remember walking beside the beach in Greece when I was 23. I was in a bikini, tanned, young, vibrant, healthy and happy. I bet I looked radiant. Three Greek men walked past and one said, "Nice face, short legs!" Fortunately I thought it was funny, but do you know, 31 years later I still remember it!

And if I am really honest, I did sometimes wonder after that if my legs were too short. Now, at 54, I really don't care and know my husband loves my legs! *I* love my legs! They work really well, are strong, are in good shape, and are the perfect length for me!

Can you transform similar experiences in your life? Can you love and accept yourself and the fact that you are doing the best you can, given all your skills and knowledge?

It doesn't matter what you do to recharge your battery and how you are generous with yourself or how you reconnect with the flow—but to reconnect is your mission for today. Make the commitment to give yourself gifts. And then make sure you receive the joy—*en*joy—every moment of it.

You deserve it.

THURSDAY: GIVE YOUR BLESSINGS

"Be generous with kindly words, especially about those who are absent."

—Johann Wolfgang von Goethe

Words are very powerful. You can bless people or destroy their spirit with words, looks and gestures.

Today is the day to look at how you use your words and nonverbals. Do you use them to bestow blessings or to criticize, belittle, drag down and destroy? Do you give people the benefit of the doubt or assume the worst?

Say or think nothing today that is not positive or kind about others—*especially* if they are not in the room. Say or do only things that lift others or situations up, or fills them with light.

Many problems, dramas and difficulties are set up in workplaces and families because people talk about others behind their back. This is so destructive, and we do it all in the name of "being objective"! No, we are not! Most of us are judging with a mean spirit, to prove we are in the right and they are the wrong.

A generous spirit will not complain, gossip and discuss flaws while another person is not there—or when they *are* there! A generous spirit looks on others with acceptance, grace and patience and does not judge. If God judged us as we judge others, and meted out blessings based on our behavior, I bet most of us would be "blessing challenged"!

I had never heard the phrase, "Bless his/her heart" before I arrived in Texas. And it took some time for me to understand that the meaning was not always literal. Avoid saying "bless his/her heart" unless you really mean it. Said without sincerity, this can be nasty, spiteful and harmful. Just because you smile as you say something nasty doesn't take away the sting.

Check your workplace and home for gossip and backbiting today. If you find it, walk away from it and choose not to be involved. (But remember, there are times when we have to do or say something to end a bad situation or protect others.) If you are the instigator of gossip or backbiting—stop! Never again are you going to gossip about or otherwise or "discuss" anyone else.

Always be a blessing to others, and if you can't, then say or think nothing harmful. Find a way to bless those around you, even if you don't like them. Ask yourself, "How could I be a blessing to . . . ?" And then do it with the right heart and generous spirit. At some level, that person deserves it, even if you *think* they don't. Maybe the blessing would be that you ask to have a meeting with the person so you can discuss "your differences" in a mature, adult way so the whole workplace (not just you two) can have more peace and harmony.

One dictionary definition of *blessing* is "something promoting or contributing to happiness, well-being or prosperity; a boon." What can you do today that will promote or contribute to someone else's happiness, well-being, prosperity, success, joy or sense of worth? How can you be a "boon" to them today? How can you help someone feel loved and love themselves better?

Ask God how you can bless others as He blesses you.

FRIDAY: RECEIVE WITH GRACE

"Human life runs its course in the metamorphosis between receiving and giving."

—Johann Wolfgang von Goethe

There are a gazillion references to receiving in the Bible. I bet it's even a law of nature to receive, accept and then bless others! If flowers could not receive the warmth from sunshine, they would not survive. If the flowers did not in turn bless the bees with pollen, the hives would not grow and so on. All cycles and rhythms would be stopped without both sides doing their part.

How are you at accepting blessings or gifts from others, from yourself and from God?

Receiving with grace means being able to accept anything given with love and allowing that love to flow into us—even if we don't feel we deserve it. Grace is an unearned gift. It comes from a Greek word, *charis* which implies a kindness bestowed upon someone that he or she has not earned.

We need to consciously live in such a way that we feel, deep down, we are loved and worthy of love. We need to feel we deserve good things and blessings in our lives.

Do you, deep inside, feel that you *don't* deserve time, gifts, acknowledgments, blessings or anything else from yourself, others and God? That you are not worthy? Be honest. Working with grace and the concept of grace is critical for learning to love and accept ourselves and others as we are. We receive His grace whether we deserve it or not.

Do you feel as if you are a one-way *stream* of giving—that everybody wants, wants, *wants* from you? Frequently, people who are very generous run into people who are very good at taking! Are you surrounded by takers, people who don't give anything in return? If you are, focus on and review the choices you have made that contributed to your situation.

Are you really being taken advantage of or have you forgotten that you offered to give initially? Or that it might be your responsibility to give as a parent, for example? Often when we feel taken advantage of, people really are trying to give to us, but we don't see that or accept it. Most people want to return generosity.

Mind you, if we are generous, there are some people out there who will knowingly or unknowingly take advantage of us. If you feel someone is taking advantage of you, you may feel resentment, and it's okay to have that feeling. It's how you *respond* to that feeling that matters. Don't withdraw immediately or do anything to harm them, but it may be a time to be cautious. Either discuss the situation with the person, or, if possible, set yourself up so that they can't take advantage of you again.

Do you ever feel love flowing into your heart, or a sense of being "bathed" in love? This can be God's grace being poured over you. I notice this the most *after* I have been giving love out to others or serving them.

Maybe you will receive intuition or inspiration or be uplifted by something that comes into your heart—these are gifts. We need to make time to receive the inspiration or intuition. Sometimes it comes in the shower—we don't even have to work at it. Only you can decide what you need to do to be able to recognize and receive love, inspiration, intuition or other forms of blessings from God and others.

Your task today is to quietly contemplate receiving and accepting love. Could you gratefully receive by sitting with God and allowing Him to fill you with His love? Or by being in nature and allowing Her to soothe your soul? Or by spending time at the ocean and feeling at one with everything?

Do you need to silence the "tormentor" in your thoughts who fills you with fear? If so, replace it with the voice of love and reason—the voice that tells you that you *are* a worthwhile person, despite what you may or may not have done.

Remember, some of God's blessings may come from other people (or angels disguised as people!) so be on the alert. You never know where or when a blessing will appear! It is *your job* to receive that blessing with grace, allow it to truly enter your heart, and *let it flow out to others*.

Of course, there are always those who bring a gift in the form of criticism. How do you receive criticism? Does it crush you or make you defensive or angry? Receiving negative comments in an adult and mature way means being able to hear them, look at them objectively, assess what truth there is in them, and then work with what you find.

Thank the person if they have opened up a valuable area of growth for you—even if it is painful. And if you find no truth in it, perhaps you can discuss it and learn to see it from their point of view.

There are blessings everywhere if you have a spirit of receiving and gratitude!

SATURDAY: **ASK AND RECEIVE**

"If ye abide in me, and my words abide in you, ye shall ask what ye will, and it shall be done unto you."

—John 15:7

Have you ever read a little book called the *Prayer of Jabez?* There was a story in there that really stuck with me.

Someone had died and was being given a tour of heaven by St. Peter. The two walked past a large building with no windows and the new-comer asked what it was. St. Peter replied, "You don't want to know." The man was insistent though, and finally St. Peter agreed to show him inside. They walked into the building, which was lined with miles of shelves. On these shelves were millions of beautiful white boxes, each tied with a gorgeous red ribbon. The man asked, "What are they?" and St. Peter replied, "They are all the blessings people never asked for while they were on earth!"

There is so much help and support available for us if only we would stop, ask and listen. Blessings come in every form you can imagine—as help, intuition, inspiration, friends, warnings, healers, surprises, money, struggles, trials, answers to hardships and great moments of joy.

Ask for all the blessings that should be yours today!

Ask, believe and you shall receive!

CHAPTER 6

A WEEK OF **FORGIVENESS**

"Forgiveness, it has to be seen, is not a one-time, one-moment act, but a spiritual path."[1]

—Robert Sardello

YOUR **SEVEN MINUTES**

Dwell for the next seven minutes on people who have hurt you, or made you angry, who annoy you and "make you crazy," whom you feel hostile or resentful towards.

At the end of this reflection, you might be a seething mass of anger, pain and other nasty emotions. That can be a good thing, because it will give you some sense of the work you need to do this week and will show you where to focus your forgiveness activities.

This week is the week you are going to start freeing yourself of the burden of resentment, anger, hostility and hurt.

And remember to forgive yourself! Most of us need to!

AMANDA'S TAKE ON FORGIVENESS

FORGIVENESS AS A WAY OF LIVING—WITH TRIFOCALS!

Joan Borysenko, a pioneer in the field of integrative medicine and the mind/body connection, once said, "Forgiveness is not a set of behaviors but an attitude." I would like to paraphrase that and say, *Forgiveness is not a set of behaviors or actions but a way of living.*

If we keep in mind what my wonderful teacher Robert Sardello says about forgiveness being a spiritual path, choosing to live "the way of forgiveness" may transform everything in your life—and maybe the world!

From now on, would you be willing to filter your life events through the lens of forgiveness? To keep with my theme—we need to wear "forgiveness" glasses *all* the time. And I believe we need trifocals! *Love* would form the outside frame and *gratitude, compassion and forgiveness* would be the three parts of the lens.

From the minute we wake up, we need to wear these glasses so we view our world through those joy and peace-enhancing filters. We would *look at* and *live in* the world with a new awareness of what is *really* going on. It's not all about us all the time! Our egos would like it to be, but it's not.

I believe our life on earth is really about loving, believing in God and the spiritual realms, and *doing* what we are meant to be doing, which is to bring the talents God gave us into being and make the world a better place. We will always be given the resources to do what we need to do if we ask and pray.

As we do things we are meant to be doing, we learn, grow, move forward and find joy.

If we just sit around and watch television, play violent video games, don't work or contribute in some way, or do only what we want, our gifts and blessings will wither, because we are not using them and contributing something to the world. We are put here to be co-creators with God—we are continually blessed for that to happen, but if we fail to understand this purpose we lose connection with our joy.

Remember that by keeping our (invisible) forgiveness glasses on, we are choosing to live more consciously, aware of all the spiritual activities that are *really* going on around us, and we understand our opportunities and responsibility to mature, make a difference and become wiser. We are less self-centered and stop seeing ourselves as helpless victims and reacting (rather than responding) to what goes on, like dandelion fluff tossed about in the wind.

Once upon a time, cultures had ceremonies to help in identifying the truth and right action. Sadly, most communities no longer support the rituals, ceremonies and sacraments that at one time pulled people together in a sort of a group intervention to facilitate forgiveness. These were rituals that would create a chance for the guilty to repent and make amends. People were enabled to move on with their lives in those societies, or at the worst, suffer banishment.

Without these societal interventions, we now have to pull out our "do-it-yourself forgiveness kits"!

In Luke 17:3, we are told, "Be on your guard! If your brother sins, rebuke him; and if he repents, forgive him." So if we see some injustice, our job is to do all we can to stop it—safely. You may have to silently forgive the transgression, but try not to let it happen again—to you or others. If someone treats you badly, it's your responsibility to tell that person they are hurting or offending you and request they stop treating you that way. This gives them an opportunity to apologize (or repent!). If they don't, you can choose to forgive them and avoid them in the future. There has to be a level of forgiveness so we can heal, but we need to take action as well.

We are not *forced* to forgive, but we have been given the *capacity* to forgive as a gift—*for us and the world.* The greatest benefit from forgiveness is to *us,* not the "forgivee"! We are not just healing ourselves when we forgive; we are helping to heal others and the world.

Rather than condemning, judging or criticizing someone, if we can say to ourselves, "There but for the grace of God go I"—or better still, "There go I"—we acknowledge we are all part of the hologram. By making the choice to forgive in whatever way we can, we are set free.

Ask God to help the people you need to forgive and to help *you* see them the way He sees them. We may not achieve it in this lifetime, but at least we can try!

The "forgivee" may not even be aware of our gracious behavior. But neither are we conscious of the grace God is continually bestowing on us without asking for acknowledgment!

LIVING FORGIVENESS

Forgiveness begins in our perceptions—our perception of what happened and our perception of whether we need to forgive or be forgiven. It's impossible to forgive without our perceptions being changed. Perceptions are the way we view and interpret reality. *Problems in life are largely about perceptions, not reality!*

With forgiveness as our way of living, all aspects of our lives might change. If someone cuts us off on the road—we can curse, shout and raise our blood pressure or we can say, "Great—an opportunity to practice forgiveness!" and smile as we look at them kindly and say, "I forgive you."

They may drive away thinking you are a jerk, never knowing they are forgiven or even that they needed to be! But *you* have normal blood pressure, can think clearly, and are less likely to go on and do something dangerous yourself.

What if someone at work does something that irritates you? Remember, you are wearing forgiveness trifocals. As soon as possible, examine your perception of the situation and then ask yourself, "Hmmm, do I choose pain, resentment and anger, or forgiveness?"

Try to see that person as God would see them, which would be with loving concern, grace, understanding and compassion. (You can throw gratitude into this mix, as the person is teaching you something and giving you a chance to practice forgiveness!)

FORGIVENESS CHANGES YOUR LIFE

"If we practice an eye for an eye and a tooth for a tooth, soon the whole world will be blind and toothless."

—Mahatma Gandhi

How great was this statement by Mahatma Gandhi and how clear was his thinking? He and the Dalai Lama are two incredibly influential people who would have more reason than most of us to be filled with revenge, anger and hostility. And what did they do? They chose the path of peace, compassion and forgiveness. And look at their accomplishments and how peace and joy accompanied them.

Revenge and resentment are destructive, and an enormous waste of time, our life forces and our energy. We only have to look at the world's wars to see what catastrophic damage they can do. Who wants a blind, toothless world? Stop it now!

When some people perceive they have been mistreated, they brood about it forever. It sits inside them festering and rotting away their insides—even after the other person dies! The brooding affects their heart, health and everything they think and do at some level. It is a continual drain on *their* life forces, not those of the one who "transgressed." Forgiveness is the only thing that will restore their health—both physical and spiritual.

It's okay, and obviously necessary at times, to feel pain, hurt and fear (which usually form the basis of anger anyway), but the sooner we choose to work *with* forgiveness, to live *in* forgiveness, the sooner we start moving out of our pain and misery. We must not feel revenge or hold grudges. Work your way through the emotions so you can arrive at forgiveness and not those other harmful states. And please, *do not infect your children with your revenge.*

If we carry these negative feelings, they grow in us. We are the ones now injuring ourselves because we are not moving on—the negativity stays on to assault us every time we think of it. This state actually casts a shadow on other aspects of our lives. How sad. We choose anger, brooding and stagnation over forgiveness, peace and movement.

Are you sensing a common theme here? Forgiveness is all about setting *you* free. The fact that it may help others and the spiritual world and heal our physical world is a side benefit!

Fear is often at the root of ongoing un-forgiveness. We say, "I will never let this happen again" as protection, and don't recognize it as the lingering fear *of a recurrence of a similar situation*—of being violated again.

We store these toxic memories and images as large and awful, and attach them to anger, outrage, hurt, pain, disappointment, fear and all the heightened emotions. We keep repeating all the language that continues to incite us, keep watching the movies in our memories, and keep the flames of anger or spears of pain alive. We need to deal with these fears. It may take some time for the toxicity of a "fresh" emotional violation to pass, but we need to let it go.

Of course forgiveness is made more difficult if it's a physical violation we've suffered, because the scarring occurs in a different way. It remains as a physical reminder of our pain. Our life path is often changed as a result, and we must rise to the occasion, overcome, and hold onto the faith that God will make it work for the good. Don't press on alone; remember, we are all part of some community. If at all possible, allow others to help, since they will grow through the process too.

Remember, the heart is an alchemical vessel. Alchemy was the birth of chemistry and originally, it was a highly spiritual profession. It is believed that alchemists did the work of transmutation—taking base metals and turning them into gold—literally, and also with significant metaphorical and spiritual implications.

The heart will transmute your emotions and turn the base metals of anger, resentment, fear and pain into the gold of forgiveness, love and freedom. If you can sincerely find your way into your heart and put the other person *and yourself* there, God/Love will heal the hurts, help you *feel* forgiveness, and change your spirit.

Your work is to make the decision to forgive and then be conscious of what, and who, you need to put into your heart.

HOW DO YOU FORGIVE? WITH ZOOTS!

So how do we find our way to our heart? By using our imagination and conscious effort.

Close your eyes and sit somewhere quietly. Focus your attention on your heart area. Now try to be inside, or put your attention on what you feel is your heart space, which may be the interior of your physical heart, the heart chakra, or the spiritual space the heart occupies.

The first time I tried to do this, at the class I mentioned earlier called "Sacred Service" (www.spiritualschool.org), I was in awe of how large my heart space seemed to be! I had no idea what to expect; I just did what the exercise was—which was to "put your attention inside your heart."

As I sat quietly and focused on the heart area, I became aware of deep silence and a vastness of space—like illuminated dark velvet. I know this might *sound* weird but it *felt* great! We all seemed to have different experiences when we did this, but we all had a sense of calm, and *felt* peace and love.

Put yourself and your own "forgivees" into your heart space and ask God or Love to help you. I imagine when I do this that God's golden white light wraps itself around both of us (or all of us if there are more!) and I stay there until I sense peace or "nothingness." It's as if everything dissolves away and all that is left is space, silence and light.

This is not always easy. It takes a considerable amount of conscious effort to keep attention focused in the heart. We have to learn to "hold" ourselves and the others in our heart while the alchemy takes place.

When my stepfather died, my mum was devastated. Some things happened that made her not only very sad but also angry. I knew that if we did not help her get past that anger, *she* would become ill. (I believe it's not *at* a period of intense stress or negative emotions that we become ill, it's about 18 months to two years *after* the intense experience that we develop cancer, rheumatoid arthritis or multiple sclerosis or have a heart attack.)

If we don't deal with our anger, hostility or grief at the time, then a seed is planted. Over the next 18 months to two years, roots and branches grow and "suddenly" there is a full-fledged disease manifested in the body from the festering and unresolved emotions. Ask people who have had a significant life-threatening event and see how many can immediately recall a prior stressful event in their lives.

Un-forgiveness has been linked with many diseases—of the body, the psyche and the spirit. In fact, there is great quote, "Un-forgiveness is like drinking poison yourself and waiting for the other person to die!" (I could not find the original source for this piece of wisdom anywhere so forgive me if it was you, and please let me know.)

I knew we had to do something for Mama, but I didn't know what until I met Dr. Paul Pearsall, who wrote a great book called *The Heart's Code*. He taught me that when we send loving thoughts to another person, not only do we boost our immune system, we also boost *theirs*. Science has proven this—it isn't space cadet stuff!

This made me think about the word, *and work* of, forgiving. The word is *for-giving*. If we are going to for-give someone, we need to *give* that person love. And if we can't bring ourselves to do it, we can ask God to do it because He loves all of us and it's easier for Him!

So I raced home to tell Mum about sending love. She was staying with me for about six weeks after my stepdad's death. I said, "Mum, we need to send love!" She, being used to me, said, "What do you mean, *send love*?"

I said, "I don't know!" because back then, I had no clue of what to do or how to do it!

We didn't talk about it anymore until it was time for her to go home. I had taken her to the airport and when I arrived home, I found a note on my pillow from Mama. She wrote how much she loved me and what a special daughter I was and wrote of many moments we had shared together. It was a wonderful note and, of course, before I had even finished reading it, I was a sobbing mess! I was full of love for my precious mum and feeling guilty because prior to reading it, I had been feeling relief that she was gone! Sorry, Mama!

At the very bottom of the note, she had drawn a great big heart on one side and on the opposite side, she had drawn another great big heart and a whole lot of little hearts in between. This was my mama's way of sending love to me.

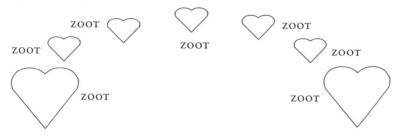

And you can do that too! Imagine little hearts going from your heart to another's. I teach audiences to do this—and we make a gesture that consists of our hands gently bouncing through the air from our heart to another's and we say the words "zoot, zoot, zoot"! Each zoot is a little heart!

So that's my mum's version of how we forgive, and how we can send love—we send zoots! She was pretty wise; she knew forgiveness happened in the heart and traveled from one heart to another. Actually, for special people she sent "zooties"!

Please teach your children this. It's a fun way to introduce what forgiveness really means and a game they'll love to play. You will be surprised at how toddlers love to zoot!

If you can't send someone "out loud" zoots, send them silently. It really does work mostly because you are changing yourself! Zoots are alchemical. But then *love* is alchemical.

FORGIVENESS AND TOLERANCE

Forgive, but don't tolerate unacceptable actions.

This was too important to leave out!

Forgiveness is so poorly understood and seems so simple that many people think they should just tolerate any kind of behavior or activity and keep forgiving. Tolerating everything can hurt *everyone*. Staying in a family situation that is abusive, or filled with pain and anger, is more likely to hurt everyone involved. After all, how can children not be affected since *everyone's* soul and spirit are connected.

Unconditionally accepting everyone does not mean having to put up with unacceptable behavior. We can, and need to, remove ourselves from that behavior, make a stand, fight it, protest against it and stop it from hurting us and others. We, with God's help and strength in our heart, can then ultimately forgive those who inflicted it—but we must not tolerate it.

A great friend of mine has learned this lesson the hard way. She is the most loving, kind person and a wonderful mother and friend. Sadly, her young adult daughter has treated her with disrespect and dishonor for a long time in many ways, but primarily by being emotionally abusive. The daughter cannot control her foul temper and speaks in an extremely offensive way to her parents. They have forgiven her repeatedly and have become resigned to the fact that this is just the way she is, which of course allows the daughter to continue this unacceptable behavior.

After a while, emotional abuse can wear people down so they tolerate any behavior—but not without cost to themselves and others. Every time this girl screams abuse at her parents, scoffs at them or treats them in some other disrespectful way, she harms their spirit. They need to take a stand, not just for themselves but also for their daughter and other children. This "tough love" might be the hardest thing they'll have to do, but it's important in order for everyone to move forward.

Forgive, but don't tolerate unacceptable actions.

PEOPLE DON'T KNOW WHAT THEY ARE DOING

"Forgive them, Father, for they know not what they do."

—Jesus Christ

For minor "misdemeanors" (as opposed to unacceptable actions), always give someone the benefit of the doubt, especially in loving relationships, unless they have given you a reason not to.

It is amazing how often we automatically assume (which makes an ASS out of U and ME) negative or harmful intentions in another. Examine your thoughts and see how often you are imagining that someone else is doing something on purpose to harm, annoy or bother you, particularly if they have not demonstrated their lack of trustworthiness in the past.

When you first meet someone, stay neutral—that is, leave expectations behind and don't look for good or bad. Discern who they really are and what their intentions might be. The difference between discerning and judging is staying neutral until you are given a clear picture of what situation and person you are really facing.

When we deal with people at a heart level, we try to trust and give them the benefit of the doubt, but it is dangerous to give a person who has bad intentions or is self-seeking the benefit of the doubt. It opens the door for their attack. We need to be discerning to receive information about their intentions and who they are.

Discernment is insight from God, and necessary. The heart has the capacity to see another person clearly, but it doesn't judge them. Being cynical, judgmental, skeptical or disbelieving is not the same as discernment. With discernment, we see things as they really are. We see the whole.

Judging others is a selfish act and unnecessary, and we only see a part of the whole when we are judging. It's finding a way to manipulate someone to do your will, your way—or putting someone down to make yourself smarter or better. Judgment is self-seeking.

TAKING OFFENSE

Think of the phrase "taking" offense. Are you someone who is offended easily—do you *take* offense at what people say or do? In that case, it's time to rethink. What's the difference between you and someone who *takes* things differently, someone who sees things in a positive or neutral light? It's *always* our perceptions—what we tell ourselves. Someone who is easily offended is often a person who is fear filled.

Unless a person is directly abusive, we would most likely "take" offense if we believed them to have negative or hurtful intentions. And we are more likely to assume everyone has those intentions if we have them ourselves!

My friend Kathy says to herself "Oh well" and moves on instead of staying hurt or angry. "Oh well" is a great phrase! Feel the initial emotions, then stop and say "Oh well" and follow it with, "Forgive them, for they know not what they do." Then move on. It makes life so much more joyful than being ambushed, kidnapped and trapped by nasty, bitter, angry, vengeful thoughts.

FORGIVE AND FORGET? OR FORGIVE AND LET GO?

> "'I can forgive, but I cannot forget,' is only another way of saying, 'I will not forgive.'"
>
> —Henry Ward Beecher

Much has been written on forgiving and not forgetting, but that phrase did not sit rightly with me. Should we forget?

We can't just obliterate something from our memory totally—it is there in the memory banks—but we can do our best not to think about it or dwell on it.

As long as the offense is not continuing, when I hear people say, "I have forgiven but not forgotten," it has a quality of "I have not really forgiven as I am still grieved by it and unhappy over it and dwell on it a lot." It feels like it would not take much to make those emotions bubble up again, as if a videotape of the offending act were being replayed continuously.

Maybe it's better to forgive and *let go*. When unforgiving thoughts come into your mind, move them, or the person, repeatedly into forgiveness (your heart) so that they can be transformed and you can truly let go. Say "Oh well" and let go!

I have had many opportunities to practice forgiveness in my life. And I have come to look at those instances as lessons that I needed to learn, and to see the people involved as just messengers. Some of them did their job very well and I am very grateful they were so diligent!

It took me some time to find a way to use these words to describe how I remember being hurt. This is very different language from the one I first used. In one particular instance, I spent a year telling everyone about what had happened to me, but each time I told the story, it stirred up pain.

I finally (DUH!) realized that I needed to stop talking about it altogether. That was when I really became conscious of the need to work on moving things to my heart, so I could forgive and let go.

Does your language keep you trapped in hurt, anger and pain? Or does it release you? Can you speak of past events in a way that brings out the blessings they ultimately brought? Or can you laugh about it? Can you see the part you played in it? Can you see the others involved in the way God would see them?

I have worked consciously on forgiveness, and when bad memories do enter my mind periodically, I use that as a reminder to work on forgiveness a little more and spend more time in my heart with those people.

FORGIVING YOURSELF—THE BIGGIE

I saved the best till last! We have talked a lot about forgiving *others* and how healing it is. Imagine if we could forgive ourselves as well.

I am so blessed that Mum taught me to not really care what other people think of me. Of course, we were taught to be respectful and do the right thing, but we were not limited by embarrassment. And I think embarrassment is a curse and a toxic emotion that gunks up your liver, shuts your soul down, and shrinks your light-filled spirit!

Everyone in my family was rather eccentric. For me, it was just a way of life to be "different" from others.

I have never felt I had to have a big fancy car or house to keep up with anyone else or prove I was as good as someone else. I bought all my furniture at the Salvation Army when I came to the U.S. and I was so proud! I felt like I was doing good while furnishing my apartment. Some people I knew were horrified, but I loved what I bought and felt good about supporting that wonderful organization.

I gave up worrying about how I looked when I was young. I had an extraordinarily beautiful and glamorous mother, as you will see from the photos, and an equally beautiful sister, and my brother was the male version of that beauty. I was told from a very young age, "Never mind, dear—you have the personality"! (Not from my mum of course, who always thought I was beautiful!)

After that, I just never worried about fussing over how I looked. I just did my best and wore what was comfortable. That's why Vermont is so perfect for me! No makeup, comfy clothes and tons of organic foods. Heaven!

Sadly, I have learned not many people were blessed with the self-confidence Mama instilled in the three of us. If we made mistakes, we learned from them and didn't beat ourselves up for being stupid. (Well, not for long anyway.) And when we had moments of embarrassment, that's all they were, moments, followed by laughter. Our behavior was not controlled by the fear of embarrassment.

Guilt was not a big issue in our family either. What is guilt, anyway? Is it really useful? I don't mean guilt over huge issues like crime, but guilt over our silly daily-life learning curves, commonly known as mistakes. Sometimes, our mistaken perceptions cause us to feel guilty, so we need to examine those and compare them with reality.

If we have done something to hurt or upset another person, or done something silly that has caused them difficulty, initial guilt can make us apologize. That is good, but then we need to let go. Guilt needs to be a gateway to responsible behavior.

Carrying guilt and embarrassment around and not doing anything to deal with them is like carrying around un-forgiveness. Self-hatred is the same, and so are all the negative thoughts we have about ourselves— "I'm a loser," "I can't do anything right," "I'm stupid" and so on. These are very victim-like statements that are not true, no matter what you say to yourself.

Challenge negative things you say to yourself and believe about yourself; they are rarely kind or true.

Take time to put *yourself* in your heart and sit there bathed in God's love. Pray for Him to help you love yourself. He loves you and so do lots of other people, so why should you not love yourself, warts and all? Send zoots to yourself!

Learn from life's lessons and let go. I love this quote from the Catholic monk Thomas À. Kempis: "Be assured that if you knew all, you would pardon all."

Forgive yourself. Forgive others. Joy will magically be with you and in you.

DAILY SCHEDULE

SUNDAY: FORGIVE THEM FOR THEY KNOW NOT WHAT THEY DO

"After all this is over, all that will really have mattered is how we treated each other."

—Anonymous

Today is the way into your future.

You are leaving the past behind and forging ahead with forgiveness as a way of living, as a spiritual path.

If anyone does anything that offends you, hurts you, disappoints you or makes you angry, think of the spiritual implications for *both* of you and use your newfound forgiveness way of living. Say "Forgive them for they know not what they do" to yourself, breathe deeply, immediately put them in your heart, and hold them there before any nasty feelings or thoughts take over.

If someone hurts you physically or is abusive, find help and, if you can, make plans to escape from this situation as soon as possible. It is unacceptable and intolerable. Then once you are safe, you can heal and work on forgiveness.

It is important to consider the right timing for forgiveness as well. Do it too quickly and you may not process the emotions adequately. If you wait too long, however, those toxic emotions will settle in and poison your liver and your soul.

There will be ample opportunities today and from now on for you to forgive. Your partner or your children will give you many reasons to practice immediate forgiveness—or better still—non-reaction! If you *respond* and don't react with anger, impatience or irritation, there is nothing to forgive in yourself—or them.

Today, nothing is going to offend you, upset you or push your buttons. You are going to breathe, stay balanced, and maintain a state of equanimity. If you slip and find you are reacting, quickly move into your heart and forgiveness then let it go.

Your new mantra is, "Forgive, let go, send love and move on!" That way you are always bringing light into the world.

MONDAY: BREAKING THE BONDS

"When you hold resentment toward another, you are bound to
that person or condition by an emotional link that is stronger
than steel. Forgiveness is the only way to dissolve that link and
get free."

—Catherine Ponder

In your seven minutes, you reflected on how you feel toward all those who have "done you wrong." When you cling to those negative feelings, whose heart, soul and spirit are being damaged? Yours.

You are, however, connected to them with a "stronger than steel" bond while you hold un-forgiveness. When we carry grudges, resentment, anger, guilt or shame towards anyone, they are living with and inside us!

Today your mission is to forgive these people. Sit quietly by yourself somewhere, make a list of them, then look at each name. Try to connect with the soul or spirit of that person—not their personality. If we can look past a personality and see more deeply into their spirit being and soul, we see a very different picture. We see their true nature, and not the selfish, egotistical, win-at-all-costs, often misguided "human" personality. We see what God sees.

After you have thought about this person and realized they did not know what they were doing, give them grace and hold them in your heart. Try to do this for at least a minute—a minute is a long time when you are doing this! Then let them dissolve into the light. Stop, breathe deeply a few times, notice how you feel, and place the next person into your heart.

When you have finished, send all of these people zoots. Try to see little zoots going from your heart to theirs. If you can't do that, ask God to sit with you and the other person and to bathe you both in His light and love. Or ask your guardian angel to help you. Maybe yours can go to the other person's guardian angel and the two of them can work out a resolution. If this sounds a little out there for you, try it anyway—you may be surprised!

TUESDAY: ASK FOR FORGIVENESS

"Finally, brethren, whatever is true, whatever is honorable, whatever is right, whatever is pure, whatever is lovely, whatever is of good repute, if there is any excellence, if anything worthy of praise, dwell on these things."

—Philippians 4:8

Ask for forgiveness—whether you did anything wrong or not!

There is a problem-solving healing process called Ho'oponopono that originated in Hawaii and has had miraculous results (www.hooponopono.org).

This process works through love. Practitioners speak of love and connecting with the original source of love, to heal the erroneous thoughts within a person that create problems for themselves and others.

The healer connects his or her heart to the Source (for me it would be God) and then sincerely apologizes for any harmful, erroneous thoughts that are within *him or her*. They apologize *to* the person, saying something like, "I am truly sorry for the erroneous thoughts I have had that have caused this problem in you and in me. Please forgive me.

These thoughts that need to be forgiven are out of alignment with the principle of Oneness and Love."

This is a stretch, I know—but I was fascinated with it and tried it. Well golly, it works! *But*—you have to really enter into the "field" of love to do it. It has to really come from deep inside your heart and you have to believe that we are all one—connected at all levels and that what *I* am thinking *does* affect *you*.

Soon after learning about this process, my husband Ken and I were driving and having a fight over navigation (as men and women in cars do!). I remembered this technique and for two hours, I repeated the above phrases. But I did it with an angry heart. I was *snarling* the words inside my head initially. (I was doing it to avoid attacking Ken!) Needless to say, that didn't work—but it was a great lesson.

Once I realized what I was doing, I dropped to my heart. I could feel the difference between saying the words from a place of real love and saying them with negative emotions.

Think about the people you believe have wronged you in the past. Now ask for their forgiveness! (I *KNOW*, you have *not done anything wrong*—but were you really totally innocent? Were you pure in all your thoughts and actions with them? Did you do *nothing* that could do with a little forgiveness? Be honest now.) Even if you were completely innocent, still ask for their forgiveness. It is part of the healing process. You don't have to ask for it out loud or in person. You can ask for it at a heart level as they do in Ho'oponopono.

It may help to sit quietly somewhere and have a picture of the person in front of you.

First, connect with God. Do nothing else until you feel the presence of love. Once you are in your heart and can really feel love, then think of the person and say, "I am truly sorry for the erroneous (or wrong or negative) thoughts I have had that have caused or contributed to this problem in you and between us. Please forgive me." (If you really wanted to make this superpowerful—you would finish with a *sincere* "I love you"!)

This only works, as I learned, if you really come from love and are sincere.

The other obvious alternative for forgiveness is to gather up your courage and character and go up to the person and ask them to forgive you. Be sincere! Or write them a note. This is also a very effective technique in most cases, but I gave you the easy way first!

WEDNESDAY: LET GO OF EMBARRASSMENT AND SHAME

> "The world, I found, has a way of taking a man pretty much at his own rating. If he permits his loss to make him embarrassed and apologetic, he will draw embarrassment from others. But if he gains his own respect, the respect of those around him comes easily."
>
> —Alexander de Seversky

Embarrassment is basically being worried about what other people think of you, isn't it? And it's often defined as "the shame you feel when your inadequacy or guilt is made public."

Note the word "your." What *you* believe to be an inadequacy or guilt is very important. It's *your* fear of *other* people's perceptions or judgments of you and what you do or have done. Ongoing shame can be reinforced by unwitting parents or friends. The shame of "not being good enough" or "as good as" someone else can control our lives and was most likely based on a false or misguided perception.

If you have respect for yourself and know your motivations and intentions to be pure and honest, why be worried what others will think? If you know you did your best, take comfort in that.

Words listed as synonyms with *embarrassment* are *chagrin, mortification, humiliation, self-consciousness, shame, being disconcerted* and *uncomfortable.* All in all, as an emotion, this doesn't seem very useful!

Today is the day for you to recall embarrassing moments and find a way to laugh at them! Explore what you were thinking at the time that made those moments embarrassing. Transform the memories with your heart—from chagrin and shame to joy in your heart. Laugh at yourself and with others!

Listen to what you say to yourself about those events. Then change your language and consciously look for the funny side. So many people waste decades being embarrassed or filled with shame—it peaks during the teenage years and some of us just don't un-peak! In my opinion, it's an unproductive use of time and means that other people will rule how you live your life.

My adored niece, Clelia, when she was nine, competed in a gymnastics competition. Since I have always been an enthusiastic person, she didn't have to do much and I would clap, cheer and jump up and down. She did her best to avoid eye contact with me, and the rest of the family stayed as far away from me as possible, but that didn't stop me!

Then I overheard Clelia say to a little friend, "She's not my mum; she's only my aunt!" I have lived off that story for years! My desire was to encourage her and show her how proud I was, out loud, and it was all done with a *sincere* heart. I figured it was good for her to see that behavior modeled, so she may feel free to do that with her own children one day. *And* she still loves me, which is most important! (Of course, I am not invited to events with her anymore! Just joking!)

Go on—be yourself—live out loud! Stop allowing your negative thoughts and the fear of what other people think or might have thought in the past to rule your behavior and life. That is what shame and embarrassment are—*belittling yourself* and letting what *others* think of you rule what you do, how you behave or how you live.

If you are enthusiastic or passionate about something, show it! If you dress differently or look at things differently from others, don't shove it down their throats, but don't deny your way of looking at the world. Whose life is it anyway?

After you have laughed at the past, make a commitment to stop your own critical, denigrating thoughts about yourself, and never let the *fear of what other people think* change or stop you from being the real you!

THURSDAY: FORGIVE YOURSELF

"The day the child realizes that all adults are imperfect, he becomes an adolescent; the day he forgives them, he becomes an adult; the day he forgives himself, he becomes wise."

— Alden Nowlan

I have already written a lot on forgiving yourself. Now is the day to do it. Forgiving yourself and loving yourself are pretty much one and the same. Remember that you were doing the best you could at the time, with the level of skills and knowledge you had. You didn't know any better, and if you had known better, you would have done something different.

Give yourself love, understanding and compassion. Imagine you are speaking to a little child that lives inside you—how would you forgive that little child? You would say to them, in a very loving way, "I know you didn't mean any harm" or "You made a mistake—that's all" or "You tried your best." They would be soothing and understanding heartfelt words. Say those things to *yourself now.*

Ask for God to help you. Put yourself in your heart and stay there until the alchemical work is done.

Continue to work on forgiving yourself, and if you can't, right a wrong elsewhere to make up for it. Sometimes to forgive ourselves, we have to make something right. If you can't make things right with the person you have in mind, then right a wrong somewhere else!

At the end of today, your goal is to have released unforgiven moments from the past, given yourself a lot of grace and love, and set yourself free to move into the future.

P.S. When we forgive ourselves, *we* need to do it whether another person has forgiven us or not. What the other person feels is of no consequence for you. You can only ask them through your heart to forgive you, then let go of whether they do or not.

FRIDAY: THE OTHER PERSON'S RESPONSE

"The other person's response doesn't matter! Forgive them whether they know you have done it or not."

—Anonymous

When we forgive others, we need to be completely unattached to the other person's response or reaction to our forgiving them. If we forgive someone else and *expect* some change from them, are we forgiving for the right reason?

Our forgiveness should be unconditional. We have made a choice to live a life of forgiveness, no matter what anyone else does or does not do or how they respond to our forgiving them!

You have already had a couple of days to practice forgiveness. Today, check to see if you are able to forgive without any expectation of what another person should or should not do. Be honest. If you are expecting something from them, stop now! Forgiveness is not true forgiveness if you expect something in return.

What is important is that *you* know you have forgiven them—and *God* knows you have forgiven them! That's all that matters. Your changed behavior and calmer nature can tell the rest of the world! And you can move on.

SATURDAY: APOLOGIZE

"Never ruin an apology with an excuse."

—Kimberly Johnson

Gulp! Apologize? Do I have to?

Well, pretty much yes, if you did something that intentionally or unintentionally hurt or harmed someone else. And as Ms. Johnson says above—never ruin it with an excuse.

If you say "I am sorry *but. . .*" you are about to make an excuse and you know you are not in your heart. It doesn't really matter why we did what we did.

By making an excuse, we are trying to justify our behavior. We are really saying with words that *sound* like an apology, "You deserved this!" or "I am not a bad person—listen to this really strong reason for my behavior that hurt you" or "It's not my fault really." Yes, it *is* our fault! We need to accept responsibility.

We always have choices in how to behave, and perhaps we chose poorly at that one point in time. We may have been tired or there may have been other extenuating circumstances, but we don't need to share them.

To apologize sincerely is to *feel* the apology in your heart first. Then and only when you *feel* true sorrow at what has happened, do you *say*, "I am truly sorry for what I did/has happened/my behavior/the pain I have caused you. Please forgive me. I will not do it again."

And then don't do it again! This is critical.

So many people apologize easily just to appease another person. They don't really feel it in their hearts, and so they continue to repeat the offending action. After this has happened a few times, an apology means nothing to the other person.

Friends of mine in Australia have a big sign above their bedroom door saying, "He who forgives first, wins!" Isn't that a great idea?

Why not make it a family activity to create and decorate several banners that say "He who forgives first, has more joy!" and then put them in prominent places in your home? It is a fun reminder of the necessity to live in a state of forgiving. Playing games with our children like this helps them comprehend what forgiveness means.

Imagine if *you* had learned at an early age how harmful anger and hostility are, and how futile and damaging revenge, resentment and grudges are. Would your life have been different if you had learned then how spectacular true forgiveness is?

Today is the day for finding those to whom you need to sincerely apologize, and doing it. Take a big breath: You will be amazed at how much better you feel at the end of the day once you have relieved your soul of these burdens you have been carrying!

What if *another person needs* to apologize to *you*? As television personality Robin Quivers once said, "An apology might help, but you can change your life without one."

No matter how much you want (or think you need) an apology from another person, you will live without it!

I had an experience of this recently, where I felt someone should apologize. They have not apologized and they will not, I suspect, but I forgave them anyway.

So how did I handle that? I asked for their forgiveness (at a heart-to-heart level—not out loud!) for my part in what had happened, even though I felt like an innocent bystander. I figured I must have had some part to play, and was sincere when I asked at that soul level for forgiveness.

I gave forgiveness at the soul level and am still working on that one to turn it from forgiveness to real love. I have held that person in my heart for at least a minute, many times, and I do feel that is working. I have asked God to help me. Once I have done the holding-in-my-heart exercise, I leave it alone and move on.

After you have apologized to all those you want to apologize to today, let go of any "needs" you have to hear an apology from them.

This could be a very freeing day!

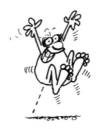

CHAPTER 7

A WEEK OF ENERGY AND VITALITY

"Aliveness is energy. It's the juice, the vitality, and the passion that wakes up our cells every morning. It's what makes us want to dance. Everything is of interest to a person who is truly alive, whether it's a challenge, a loving moment, a bucket of grief, or a glimpse of beauty."[1]

—Daphne Rose Kingma

YOUR SEVEN MINUTES

Do you wake up every morning full of energy and vitality?

Do you go home every night full of energy and vitality?

Or do you just want to remember what it felt like to *have* energy and vitality?

Reflect on all the things that give you energy and make you feel alive. Are they things such as exercise, sleep, relaxing, learning and laughing? Spending time doing something you love? Are there certain people who energize you?

What or who seems to drain your energy?

At what time in your life did you have a lot of energy and vitality? What was your joy level at the time?

AMANDA'S TAKE ON ENERGY AND VITALITY

"You only lose energy when life becomes dull in your mind. Your mind becomes bored and therefore tired of doing nothing. Get interested in something! Get absolutely enthralled in something! Get out of yourself! Be somebody! Do something."

—Norman Vincent Peale

Energy and vitality are signs of total wellness—that our whole being feels really alive—vibrating with God's love. Anything that brings us closer to God or the Divine brings us joy and makes us feel alive.

How many times have you felt exhausted and drained and then found new energy doing something fun, or something meaningful? The spirit in which we act affects our vitality levels; a positive and enthusiastic spirit charges us with light and life forces. So even in a busy, rushed lifestyle, we can find joy if we have the right spirit.

If we are exhausted or disconnected from God and ourselves, we may find moments of joy in a beautiful scene, a child who hugs us or a partner who reassures us, but *maintaining* that state of joy is more difficult.

We *are* spiritual beings in a human body. Our body is the "temple" for our spirit (or the Holy Spirit, as the Bible says), and our responsibility is to take care of the temple. Therefore we must be conscious of how we treat our physical body.

This chapter is focused on physical energy and has many lessons from my own experiences when my "temple" was in bad shape, although I do practice what I preach—or try to!

If you are not as well as you wish to be, I would encourage you to explore what has *really* robbed you of your vitality or brought ill health—whether it is physical, emotional, psychological or spiritual.

DEPRESSION AND EXHAUSTION OR
LYME DISEASE AND CELIAC DISEASE?

I used to have incredibly high energy levels. I would make people exhausted just describing what I did during a day—and I had fun! And then I spent four years still doing a lot but feeling exhausted most of the time.

I looked okay—tired but okay. I was crabby and if I didn't sleep ten hours a night, I had no energy. My relationship suffered because there was nothing left for my long-suffering husband at the end of dragging myself through one of my busy days.

As many doctors I visited told me, I had plenty of reasons to be tired. I traveled a huge amount and had been through a very stressful event before I left Australia. My mother was ill and I was away from her and unable to help much. I was living in a new country where I knew very few people. And I was in love with a man who lived in Australia!

All in all, it was easy and accurate for doctors to tell me my adrenals were exhausted. But that was not the whole story.

The adrenal glands sit on top of the kidneys and secrete a lot of stress-related hormones. When we stay under stress for long periods, they fatigue, cannot function properly and basically mess up most of our body physiology, balance and functioning. There are many books written on this topic because so many women (and these days, men) have problems with their adrenal functioning.

The treatment is to relax, slow down, do less, eat better, sleep and do all those healthy things that you would be doing if you had time. But since you can't stop your life to that degree, the condition worsens.

I did as much as I could and it made no difference. Then I found a fabulous naturopathic doctor in Dallas who believed I had adrenal exhaustion but saw it as a symptom and not the cause of my run-down state.

LYME DISEASE—A CLEVER SUPERBUG

The real cause of the problem was Lyme disease, which comes from a bacteria most commonly transmitted by ticks, fleas and mosquitoes. I had it in combination with Epstein-Barr, the type of virus that causes infectious mononucleosis for many adolescents and young adults. These two conditions had led to all my other problems.

I am not a physician or a medical expert, but I can share with you my personal experiences. This knowledge and blessed insight from Dr. Jim Lane of Dallas, my naturopath, and Mary Forte, a master herbalist, led me to explore Lyme disease and learn more about it.

I started to realize just how many symptoms I had experienced over the years that now made sense—jaw pain, back pain, irritability, shoulder pain, loss of memory, failing eyesight, very dry skin, depression, zero libido and exhaustion, to name a few!

The best book I have found on this subject is *Healing Lyme* by Stephen Harrod Buhner. (He is brilliant and so is the book.) Following Buhner's protocol, and the wonderful advice and treatment of Dr. Jim and of my friend Mary, has me feeling 200% better!

I learned that Lyme disease can mimic about 300 other diseases, many of them neurological, and it affects a huge number of people in the world today. Unfortunately, it is not often recognized *because it mimics* all those other diseases and is misdiagnosed.

Symptoms can affect any tissue, organ or joint in the body. Lyme spirochetes are clever little spiral-shaped bacteria that do not just live in the blood—they also burrow into individual cells. I had them in my eyes, bladder, skin, uterus, brain, nervous system, joints and probably every-where else. In retrospect, I actually don't know how I kept going.

Those who are doing the research into Lyme disease claim it has reached epidemic proportions in the U.S. and is rapidly spreading. Lyme disease is not just spread by ticks but also by mosquitoes and fleas, and some people believe it can be spread person to person. Fibromyalgia, lupus, chronic fatigue, multiple sclerosis and ALS are just some of the diseases that experts believe Lyme can mimic. If you feel unwell and in your heart you think you have not discovered the true cause of your symptoms, have a test for Lyme disease.

It is quite difficult to test definitively for Lyme disease, but I found one place that I believe really gives you the best chance of finding it. At Bowen Research & Training Institute Inc., located in Palm Harbor,

Florida, physician Dr. JoAnne Whitaker is conducting ongoing research into this subject. (She had Lyme disease herself, which has motivated her to do the research. Visit www.centralfloridaresearch.com.)

I was tested through them and was very impressed with their thoroughness. Ask your doctor to arrange for this particular test.

If you want to do some of your own research on this subject, visit www.samento.com and also www.neuraltherapy.com for information from Dr. Deitrich Klinghardt, M.D., PH.D., board-certified in neurological and orthopedic medicine. He is founder and president of the American Academy of Neural Therapy. (You can also contact me at amandagore@earthlink.net for details on great people who might be able to help you.)

On a related note, since I believe it's more difficult for us to pursue joy if we constantly feel exhausted, I'd like to mention another condition called celiac disease. I am not an expert on this but would like to share some of what I have learned.

If you have not heard of this term, it refers to an allergy to gluten. That may ring a bell, but if not, it's worth reading the book *Dangerous Grains* by James Braly and Ron Hoggin to find out just how many people are actually allergic to grains and pasteurized dairy products. It may include you!

As with Lyme, the symptoms of celiac disease are many and varied, but all result in your digestion and intestines being severely damaged.

When someone is allergic to gluten—which, by the way, is in almost every processed product—they lack certain enzymes necessary for their bodies to digest the large protein that is called gluten. Most celiacs don't have the enzymes to digest casein, either, which is the protein in dairy products.

As a result of the lack of this enzyme, the large gluten molecules leak across the gut walls into the blood. This continual leaking eventually destroys the gut lining, with pretty bad health consequences.

Having large proteins floating around in the blood is not so great either, since the immune system may see them as foreign invaders and attack them. This can lead to many other symptoms that mimic many other diseases.

Gluten sensitivity can cause an array of symptoms such as irritable bowel syndrome, gas, bloating, pain in the stomach, aches and pains, malnutrition, mood swings, aggression, depression, anxiety (very common), autoimmune disorders and mental illness.

There are definitive tests that will tell you quickly if you are allergic to gluten and casein—you may need to ask your doctor to have them done.

Some believe there are genetic factors that predispose a person to celiac allergy, so if your baby does not respond well to flour and products with gluten in them, it would be worth checking to see if they lack the necessary enzymes.

One way you may be able to test for this is an elimination diet, which means you stop eating all gluten and dairy for a month or so. If you are allergic, you will notice pretty rapid changes in how you feel. Go off every little bit of those proteins for at least a month and then test yourself—eat some gluten and see what happens.

Gluten is in all products containing wheat and is in oats, rye and barley. That means to be gluten free, you cannot eat breads, cookies, muffins, wheat pasta, cereals or anything else made with those products—unless it is gluten-free. Be careful with sauces, relishes, condiments and soups as well. Read all the labels. Luckily, many books have been written on gluten-free cooking, and more gluten-free products are available in health-oriented supermarkets.

It is believed that there is no safe level of gluten if you are allergic to it.

There are other things that may sap your energy and vitality. You really know all about them, which is why I spent so much time writing on what you may not know! We all know that exercise, adequate sleep, good food, good eating habits and balanced lifestyles, rhythms and routines are all critical for energy and vitality. We just don't do them! We work too much, travel too far, rush when we eat, don't balance work with play, are too stressed and so on, and then we wonder why we don't feel good!

Below are some simple ways to establish healthy routines that can restore some of your energy and vitality from a physical perspective.

DAILY SCHEDULE
SUNDAY: **SPIRITUALLY REENERGIZE**

"The more you lose yourself in something bigger than yourself, the more energy you will have."

—Norman Vincent Peale

This is the day to tap into the giant "battery" in the sky or all around you. Make a commitment to find your spiritual renewal center—it's really inside you, not outside!

Be quiet and spend time with God, or whatever spiritual source you believe in, or be in nature. Spend time with children—yours or someone else's. Whenever my hussband and I play with our godchildren, we go home physically tired but spiritually renewed and energized. We love spending time with them.

Contemplate, meditate, sit in silence and allow the silence to gently seep into your soul. Try talking to God like He's a person sitting with you—He really is!

If you don't know how to meditate, you can simply sit and pray. (*Kneeling* and praying is even better!) Or sit in a quiet spot on your own and focus on nothing but your breathing. Imagine your breath flowing in and out of your heart area. Or instead of focusing on your breathing, you can find a sound that relaxes you—perhaps *ah* or *om* or whatever sound you like that works for you.

Your mind will wander to other thoughts, but just gently bring it back to your focus. The mind is designed to think, so it is almost impossible to stop it. However, we can train it to rest every so often!

Try to make a time every day at the *same time* so that you do this for five to seven minutes. You can spend longer if you wish—20 minutes a day is great! Some days you may need longer than other days.

For me, slowing down and truly feeling *God's* presence is what really recharges me. I can't always do it, but I practice regularly. More often, I find the silence and just sit in it. Robert Sardello's book *Silence* (www.spiritualschool.org) might help you with this—it helped me!

Take the time today to do something that lets your soul rest and your spirit renew. Stop rushing, make some time for peace, and enjoy the renewed sense of gentle energy that comes to you.

MONDAY: EATING AND DRINKING PATTERNS AND ROUTINES

"The secret of your future is hidden in your daily routine."

—Mike Murdoch

The body renews itself on a regular basis using building materials directly derived from what we put into it. We become what we eat, so what you put into your body should be very carefully selected—it will become part of you soon!

If you buy processed foods, you may be compromising your health every time you eat them. I know you have heard of the dangers of trans fatty acids, excessive sugars and salts in most processed foods, and high-fructose corn syrup, which is in almost every premade product. You may have seen articles on artificial sweeteners, flavors and colors and what they do to us.

Pay attention to these warnings. They are not written by people who want to destroy you, but rather your habit of eating and drinking substances that can harm you.

Today is the day to observe your eating, shopping and drinking patterns and routines. Where do you shop? Do they have good, fresh foods? Do you look at the *ingredient list* on *every* processed item you buy?

Do you prepare and cook food yourself or just buy it all pre-prepared? Do you buy organic or local fresh food when you can? Organic foods are grown without pesticides. Pesticides are toxic and are usually on, or in, the fruits and vegetables we buy—wash any item very thoroughly if it is not organic. Root vegetables and potatoes absorb pesticides in the soil so try to at least buy organic potatoes and root vegetables this week, and from now on if you can.

If you live largely on processed foods, try to change this pattern. It may take more time to buy fresh food and cook it, but you will feel better; bond with your family more (especially if you make mealtimes a family affair!); teach your children how to cook; give your kids a better start in life; and be planting the seeds for a much healthier old age for them—and you.

What about lunch—can you find a place that makes organic salads or sandwiches? Try to avoid eating the potato chips that come with sandwiches and ask for fruit instead. Can you make something healthy at home the night before and take this for lunch? Or take leftovers from dinner and save money?

SNACKS

If you snack during the day—do you really need to? And if you must, on what do you snack? Every mouthful you eat can either be beneficial or harmful. Do you choose candy or cookies? Or do you choose fruit and protein bars with the least amount of sugar you can find, fresh nuts and seeds (walnuts are great!), and vegetable sticks?

Think about what you drink during the day. Is it water, a caffeinated drink or soda? Most of us are chronically dehydrated—we need to drink more water, especially if we live in air-conditioned spaces. Put some lemon or lime wedges in your water if you want flavor!

Do you live on coffee and sodas at work? If you must have something hot, try tea. Buy your own herbal teas so you can enjoy more variety in flavors. It is suspected that problems start when people consume several caffeinated drinks a day. Apart from coffee or tea, there are other sources of caffeine like standard sodas and energy bars, so be conscious of how much caffeine you really are taking in. If you go off caffeine and have withdrawal signs, you were probably having too much!

Squeeze your own juices or visit a juice bar—vegetable juices work wonderfully to renew energy.

HOW WE EAT

Also have a look at *how* you eat. If you are shoving your food down in a hurry while you're typing, writing or driving, your body cannot really digest it in the optimal way.

We need to have little rituals while we eat: Stop. Sit. Bless the food. Eat it slowly, and chew each mouthful 30 times. Yes, 30 times! Try doing that and you'll see you don't really chew your food *at all*. You may not even be aware that you shove your next mouthful in before you have swallowed the previous one.

Chewing 30 times allows the sensory systems set up in the mouth to prepare the stomach and digestive system for the food that is about to arrive—the process triggers the release of the appropriate digestion enzymes. (Ideally, we should not watch television either while we eat—especially if the show is violent or gruesome, because that is sure to affect our digestion!)

Avoid drinking water while you are eating since this dilutes your digestive juices and interferes with healthy digestion.

Many of the bad eating and drinking habits we have are just that—habits. Once we can see the patterns or rituals we are stuck in, we can change them! We can create new rituals and patterns that help our digestion and health.

Here's a great strategy: Ask yourself, "Does my health want this or my mouth (or appetite)?" Very often it's thirst or our *taste* buds that trigger our desire to eat. Stop and decide whether it's a stomach need or a mouth need or try drinking a glass of water, and you may be able to put off eating something unhealthy.

Do something to make your food exciting—to create an appetite! Set the table beautifully. Present the food so it looks wonderful on the plate. Have an excited attitude as you present the food. When possible, involve your family so they enjoy the preparation of the food. Let them be involved in some of the decision-making process—make it a fun event. Create, today, a new and much healthier rhythm and routine of eating and drinking for you and your family.

P.S. Remember to prepare your food with love! What you are feeling and thinking as you prepare food can make its way into the final product! Try to be in a loving state and be thankful for the food as you prepare it. Say grace and thank God for your food and ask Him to bless it.

We may not be able to scientifically prove that these things make a difference, but I bet we will one day!

TUESDAY: BE CONSCIOUS OF WHAT YOU DRINK

Water is essential for life. The average adult body is 55% to 75% water. Two-thirds of your body weight is water. Make sure you drink enough good-quality water!

It is amazing how quickly the body can dehydrate. By the time we actually feel thirsty, we are probably already dehydrated. Most of us are frequently dehydrated and don't even know it. It is better to drink small amounts of water every 30 minutes (apart from when you are eating) instead of drinking a full glass twice a day!

And often when we feel hungry, we are actually thirsty. Next time you feel hungry, have a glass of good-quality spring water and see what happens to your hunger. (Or just drink tap water that has a filter for fluoride and chlorine removal.)

In America and most Western countries, tap water is usually germ-free *but* we do need to consider using a good-quality filtering system to remove the chlorine and fluoride. You may want to do a search on the web and read about the potentially harmful effects of long-term sodium fluoride (added to water and toothpaste) ingestion. Some people believe sodium fluoride does not protect your teeth and does not keep your bones strong—and instead that it often has the reverse effect! It's believed that *calcium* fluoride, as it occurs in vegetables like cauliflower, is extremely beneficial to bones and teeth.

If you are thinking, "I drink a lot of sodas and coffee and tea, so I can't be dehydrated," you may be wrong! Did you know that the average American drinks *52.9 gallons* of carbonated soft drinks (full of high-fructose corn syrup or artificial sweeteners) a year? That might provide liquid but it's not like pure spring water!

Caffeine is dehydrating, apart from all the other things it does to your body. Why do you think people have withdrawal symptoms such as headaches and behavior changes and bad moods when they suddenly stop drinking a lot of coffee and soft drinks?

If you want to drink a lot of something other than water, there are many benefits in green tea. Find an organic green tea that you like and drink it when you feel like a break from water. I figure if we bless our food before we eat, why not bless our water as well!

Do you know that one of main ingredients by far in an average soda is high-fructose corn syrup (HFCS)? It is not natural fructose—it is highly processed and comes from corn. Research is showing that HFCS is associated with obesity. In an article in the *Seattle Times* (December 4, 2005), Dr. George Bray was quoted as saying, "High-fructose corn syrup isn't completely responsible for the nation's 6 million overweight children" but "it's a big part of the problem." Do yourself a favor and learn more about HFCS—it's in almost every processed food item you buy.

Please think twice before you drink ordinary sodas! Keep them out of your home and teach your children to drink water or natural juices. There are some sodas available at the health food store or in the health section of your supermarket that contain natural fruit juice sweeteners or evaporated cane juice. Read your labels carefully—and remember "natural" on the label does not always mean the same natural we are imagining!

And before you breathe a sigh of relief, thinking, "I drink *diet* sodas," know that there are many who believe diet drinks to be equally bad! Diet drinks have artificial sweeteners that are *ARTIFICIAL!* Warning!!

You may want to read *Sweet Deception* by Dr. Joseph Mercola or *Aspartame Disease: An Ignored Epidemic* by H. J. Roberts for more scientific details that may convince you to change your habits.

Today is the day to start drinking more water, preferably spring water or filtered tap water—a mouthful or two every 30 minutes—and blessing it before you drink!

WEDNESDAY: BE CONSCIOUS OF HOW MUCH YOU MOVE

We live in a society where people are searching for artificial energy-boosting substances when just doing some physical activity every day may provide that extra push to make it through the day.

Go through a typical day in your mind from the minute you wake up to when you go to bed. How much do you move? Is going from chair to chair your primary source of movement? Do you stand on escalators rather than walking up them? Do you drive when you could walk; take the elevator when you could use the stairs; send emails to the person across the floor rather than walking over to them?

What do you do when you arrive home? Do you do active or vigorous housework or have you hired a cleaner and a gardener to save you the effort of moving?

Think about your posture at work and at home. Do you slouch over your desk? Do you ever stand and stretch? Do you have pain in your neck, shoulders or low back? These are often caused by your posture and lack of movement and are warning signs that you need to move!

Think very honestly about your movement levels during the day—it may save you years of pain later.

The vast majority of us have become sedentary. We don't notice how little we move in front of and from our computers, or how we use email to send notes to each other rather than getting up and (gasp) making human contact! Or we text message from one room to another!

And *walk* to the store? Are you kidding!

The human body *must* move. *Everything* stops working well when we stop moving. You only have to see the effect paralysis has on muscles, digestion, metabolism and joints to understand that. Movement to joints is like spraying the lubricant WD-40 into them! If we don't stretch and use our muscles, we end up old, stiff and stuck when we are still young.

I am 54 and my joints are almost as flexible as they were when I was 20—and that is the way it is meant to be. I don't have a special body that is more elastic than everyone else's. I have just kept mine moving.

I have done yoga for years—and not fancy stuff. I just do eight exercises a day. I stay active and am conscious most of the time of my posture. (And my husband's! It drives him nuts, but he will thank me when we are both 90 and still active.)

As a physical therapist, I saw thousands of people with pain—and the vast bulk of it was caused by their inactive lifestyles. People in their seventies and eighties are often frail and fall because their muscles are weak and they shuffle. I am on a campaign to keep everyone strong before shuffling sets in!

Our former next-door neighbor in Dallas is a lovely, active 83-year-old. She lives on her own and is amazing. Recently, she had to stop walking on her beloved bird trails because of pain in her knee. Out of desperation, she started going to aerobics and weights classes. She is a new woman! She says she feels so much better, has no pain and has a new lease on life. That's what exercise and strengthening work does—at any age. (Of course, you need to check with your doctor before you embark on an exercise program.)

From the age of 45, we really need to be building up our muscles. Of course we also need aerobic work as well—but with age we need both. Sorry!

But wait, there's more! We need to build movement into our daily lives at the very least. I sit on a big exercise ball when I work because it makes me move more than a chair. (Be careful if you decide to do this that you are stable and that the ball will not roll away from you!) And I make sure I stand and stretch every 30 minutes.

Will you do that? Just stand up and stretch as much as you comfortably can—just for a minute—that's all. It can be for a very short time but it has a great effect on your body and your energy levels.

Can you use the stairs at work instead of the elevator or escalator? Can you park the car farther away and walk in safety? Can you go for a walk at lunchtime instead of swapping one seat for another as you eat? Can you play a game with your children instead of *all* of you sitting in front of a television? Walk daily if your neighborhood is safe. If not, can you run up and down your stairs at home for 20 minutes? (Check with the doctor before you start if you are not used to exercise.) Can you buy a treadmill? Or clean the bathroom or kitchen vigorously?

There are many ways to bring movement into your home and workplace. Be creative and find as many as you can. Your energy levels will skyrocket if you make movement and exercise a part of your daily—or even weekly—routine.

But wait, there's even more!

Exercise is also the best way to bust stress—and pain! If you feel burning, tingling, tightness, stiffness, numbness, heaviness, dragging, discomfort and pulling anywhere, your body is screaming out—*MOVE!* These are the warning signs of impending damage. If we feel pain, it's usually too late and the damage is done. So listen to your body and stretch it more.

Think for a moment how seldom children sit still for long periods; they are forever moving and playing. Limit the time your children spend mesmerized in front of the television or the computer. These are things that can stop a child from doing what they innately know is critical—moving!

Today is the day to make movement and exercise a regular routine in your life and your family's life.

THURSDAY: SLEEP AND ENERGY

"Lack of sleep disrupts every physiological function in the body.
We have nothing in our biology that allows us to adapt to
this behavior."[2]

—Eve Van Cauter

"People who are sleep-deprived have elevated levels of substances
in the blood that indicate a heightened state of inflammation in
the body, which has recently emerged as a major risk factor for
heart disease, stroke, cancer and diabetes."[3]

—Dr. Sanjay R. Patel

Exercise is critical for our health, energy and vitality, and so is sleep.

While we sleep, we heal and recharge our batteries, yet gazillions of people are not sleeping well, partly because we are not exercising enough to make us physically tired!

Instead, we exercise our minds all the time and rarely let them rest, and so we are constantly feeling stressed. That means we go to sleep exhausted and then find ourselves wide awake at 3 a.m.!

How are your sleep patterns? Generally, to be well, we need about seven hours of sleep a night, which is hard if you have young children, I know! Do you wake up refreshed and alert? If not, here are a few tips:

Try to exercise sometime during the day so you have some real physical fatigue—not just mental exhaustion. If you are going to exercise at night, do it before dinner so that you are not energized just before you go to sleep. Do not take your laptop or any work to bed! That will probably make you stay up much later than you planned and stimulate your mind just before sleeping.

Avoid watching television in bed. Watching anything other than a meditation channel with soft music and beautiful scenes is unlikely to help you sleep! Instead of zoning out in front of the television, try lying in bed and reading an inspirational book until you fall asleep. You might be surprised at how much of a difference this makes.

Listen to beautiful, relaxing music just before you sleep or as you are falling asleep. Try a meditation tape or a tape of music designed to make you sleep—there are many available. Try to make the room as dark and as quiet as possible.

If you don't want to read, climb into bed and quietly reflect on the day, focusing on things for which you are grateful. Allow in only thoughts of gratitude.

Perhaps you can take notes on these thoughts.

Always have a notepad and pen by your bed. Often when we wake up and can't go back to sleep, it's because we have thought of some brilliant idea and we stay awake (even unconsciously) because we are concerned we will forget it. Or we wake up and think of some problem that is bothering us, but if we write it down, we can tell ourselves we will worry about it tomorrow at a better time. And that often lets us go back to sleep.

Sometimes before we go to bed, making a list of all the things we have to do the next day helps the mind shut off and lets peaceful sleep drift in. Actually, it's better timing to do this just before you leave work in the afternoon!

Sometimes, if you write down a problem before you go to sleep and ask God to provide you with a solution, you will be amazed at how the answer is there when you wake up. Or it may come to you in the shower! It's wonderful how often this works, as long as you let the problem go once you have written it down and trust the answer will come.

If you wake up and can't go back to sleep, try focusing on your breathing. Just imagine the breath flowing in and out of your lungs or heart area gently and rhythmically. Maybe imagine a color with it as well. Or create the feeling that you are floating on a huge, very still lake—you are safe, protected and fully supported as you completely relax into the feeling of the lake.

If possible, try to set up a rhythm and a set of rituals for going to bed. Aim to go to bed at the same time each night—the earlier the better. Some people say that every hour of sleep before midnight is worth two after midnight! Perhaps you can have a warm bath or shower as part of the ritual before you go to bed. Talk about only positive things—not about all your worries and problems. Maybe you and your partner can give each other a massage once a week.

You may wish to pray (on your knees or not) for a few minutes each night just before you sleep. Allow God to hold you and comfort you. Praying for those you love, then counting your blessings and dwelling on gratitude to God is one of the best ways I know to go to sleep!

Sometimes what we eat before we sleep can make a difference. For example, bananas have magnesium and serotonin; chamomile tea has a mild sedative effect; warm milk, almonds and slices of whole wheat toast actually contain tryptophan, which relaxes us; and a tiny bit of raw honey helps too.

Listening to what we say to ourselves as we go to sleep and staying away from the television and computer for at least an hour before bed may be the only things we need to do to transform our sleep and allow us to wake up feeling refreshed and alert.

And speaking of waking up—try to find an alarm that does not cause you to sit bolt upright in bed with terror! A gentle welcome into the day is much better than the sudden jarring that many alarms provide.

Today—prepare to sleep well and make this your new rhythm.

FRIDAY: **BUST STRESS**

Stress is a fact of life but it doesn't have to be a way of life!

Stress is probably the greatest zapper of energy and vitality. Constant stress and pressure are exhausting both mentally and physically. Remember your adrenal glands and how hard they work when you are stressed.

Today, do your best to stay calm and peaceful. Watch carefully what you say to yourself, *as most of our stress comes from our words and perceptions.*

Listen carefully to your internal dialogue or self talk and challenge the truth of it. Events that happen are just events. They are neither good nor bad, but we perceive and *judge* them as good or bad. For example, if we see a strange look on our boss's face, we suddenly fear we might have done something wrong, when really the boss may have just had a moment of indigestion!

If you worry a lot, think about the value of worrying. Will it change things? Probably not, but you will waste a lot of time and energy. If you are con-cerned and take action to rectify the situation, you won't waste time stewing in worry and not doing anything! Try saying "Oh well." I have found many times that if I say "Oh well" I breathe again and relax.

Which brings me to breathing. *Deep* breathing is probably the greatest weapon against stress!

When we feel stressed, our breathing becomes shallow and rapid. There is less oxygen delivered to the brain and we stop thinking clearly.

Notice your breathing today and keep taking deep, long breaths in and *out*. It's often the out breath that suffers when you are stressed. Breathe out all the bad stuff!

Can you make a commitment today to avoid all rushing? Sometimes we are so in the habit of rushing we have no idea why we are racing around our house! Wake up earlier if you need more time to do what you need to do. Leave the house a little earlier so you are not driving like a crazy person, creating even more stress for yourself and others.

Breathe deeply, slow down and stop all stress-inducing self talk, and you may be surprised at how calm you stay and how much more alive you feel at the end of the day.

SATURDAY: ENERGY GIVERS AND SUCKERS

"Don't hold onto your anger, hurt and pain. They steal your energy and keep you from love."

—Anonymous

Have you ever woken up feeling pretty energetic and then encountered someone who leaves you feeling completely drained in only five minutes? These people are real and I call them energy suckers. They are psychic vampires!

I bet at some stage in your career, you have had someone on your team like this. What was it like when they left? It seemed as if the sun had come out! Everyone was laughing, working well together and happy all of a sudden!

That's the impact an energy sucker can make in your life, at home or at work. *One* energy sucker can destroy a very large team! Typically they are pessimists and cynics, and they think they are superior. They often put people down to make themselves feel better.

Avoid them like the plague! Do everything you can to limit your time and exposure to these people. If you have to be around them, try to prepare yourself. Imagine there is a cocoon of armor or light or some impenetrable material around you. You can give energy out of this cocoon, but no one can take it out without your permission. This sounds silly but it is pretty effective!

If you live with an energy sucker, try the cocoon. You can also show them the DVD I have available on my website describing the difference between energy givers and suckers and hopefully they will get the hint! Try to counteract the time you have to spend with these energy suckers by hanging around lots of energy givers.

Energy givers are happy, optimistic, upbeat, positive people and they always make us feel better. Hang around them as much as you can. Try to *be* one as well. Do the things in this book and you automatically *become an energy giver!*

It's a parent's job to teach children optimism. But because we don't consciously focus on teaching children optimism, we often model energy-sucking ways for them. And then we wonder why some, or all, children are little energy suckers!

Be cheerful and focus on helping children (and yourself) see the bright side of life rather than the rush, frustration, anger and disappointment. They will have plenty of time to learn that themselves when they are older.

Today is the day you are to make your home a haven for energy givers. Banish energy suckers! Be positive and optimistic, and play and have fun with your family. Laugh a lot.

Be the CEO–the chief energy officer!

CHAPTER 8

A WEEK OF **LISTENING**

"God gave us two ears and one mouth. He was hinting."

—Anonymous

YOUR SEVEN MINUTES

Are you a good listener? If you asked the people in your family, what would they say? What would your colleagues at work say and your friends? Be honest!

What person in your life listens to you the best? What do you experience when they are listening intently? How do you feel afterwards? Can you determine what happens during the experience that invokes those feelings?

Think of a person you know who really does not listen at all. Or someone who interrupts you all the time. What is it like to be around them? How do you feel? Where is that feeling in your body?

AMANDA'S TAKE ON LISTENING

"Conversation: a vocal competition in which the one who is catching his breath is called the listener."

—Anonymous

LISTENING VS. HEARING

Very few people are great listeners. Or even good listeners! Listening and hearing are completely different. Most of us can hear—but how many of us really listen?

Do you remember a very touching song by Mike and the Mechanics called "In the Living Years"? It was about the conflicts in communication between a father and his son. The chorus has a line, "You can listen as well as you hear." This really struck a chord with me.

Another anonymous quote says, "Hearing is a faculty; listening is an art." Dictionary definitions of "hearing" are mostly linked to the actual physical ability to hear. We are either capable of hearing or not. We hear sounds but we have to listen for meaning. More importantly, we listen for feelings. We sort through the sounds to discover what the person's soul or heart is saying.

When we truly listen, we pay attention to far more than just words. We see the body language; we pay attention to the voice tones (these are very powerful, as my husband will tell you!); we watch facial movements and expressions, breathing and eye movements. We tune in to every little nuance. We set aside our own thoughts and chatter. We see the world through the other person's eyes—and feel their soul. We can actually understand what they are saying because we are entering their reality.

Hearing is easy for most of us. Listening takes work.

LISTENING AND THE HEART

"Words are just words, and without heart they have no meaning."

—Chinese proverb

Hearing is a faculty of biology. Listening is a quality of the heart. That means we *must be "in our hearts" to really be listening*.

If we are doing other things while someone speaks, we are just hearing sounds. Unless we are totally focused on them, we cannot enter their reality/world and see things the way they see them, which is the only way we can understand how someone else might feel.

Have you ever been driving with a child in the back of the car and they are babbling away about some important story (for them) to which you respond with all sorts of "uh-huh" noises. Finally the little one says, "Mommy/Daddy, you're not listening to me!" And they are right!

Hearing, without the quality of listening, never enters the heart or soul, and people sense this, especially children.

When someone speaks, there are the words, and then there are the other dimensions of actual communication.

When people talk, they also use their faces, bodies, voice tones, breathing, pauses and other nonverbal qualities. These nonverbal cues are the second dimension of communication. The third and probably most important dimension is that which comes from their heart and soul. These are much gentler, subtle vibrations. They can only be picked up with a heart that is tuned in.

Feelings come wrapped in words, tones and nonverbal gestures. It's the *feeling* people want us to respond to, not the words, and yet most of us are unconscious of those wrapped, tender feelings!

We hear their words, wait for the next gap in the conversation and jump right in with our own words. Those of course wrap around *our* feelings, which we want *them* to respond to, but the other person does not "see" or sense our feelings and so the loop continues. And we both end up unheard and unhappy.

Imagine what would happen if *every* time you listened to someone, you were really aware that these words were just wrappings around feelings. That is being-in-the-heart listening!

This may be alchemical! Transformational!

Listening is very active and is something that takes concentration and effort. You are hearing, unwrapping, going to your heart and decoding. There is a lot to do when you truly listen; you can't be busy doing something else or planning your return volley of words.

Stephen R. Covey says in his book *The Seven Habits of Highly Effective People,* that "Most people do not listen with the intent to understand; they listen with the intent to reply. They are either speaking or preparing to speak." That leads him to one of his golden rules: "Seek first to understand, THEN be understood."

If we can do this, we are in our hearts and truly listening.

WE CAN'T FAKE LISTENING

When there is a really important conversation you need to have (all of them are really!), take time initially to go into your heart. If you can be in your heart the whole time you listen, it is easier to understand what the other person is really trying to say. They will feel heard and acknowledged. Conversely, they *will also sense* when you are judging what they are saying, preparing your "defense" or waiting for them to stop speaking so you can burst forth with what you have been preparing to say!

Mother Teresa said, "We need silence to be able to touch souls." If we are going to touch someone else's soul through listening, and really have them *feel* heard, acknowledged and validated, we need to be in a *state* of silence while we listen to them—and this does not just mean there is no sound coming out of you or anyone else! It means there is a deep silence within your heart.

Very often, true listening involves making noises that indicate you are *with* the person speaking and following what they are saying. And these shouldn't be just "uh-huh" noises to make them *think* we are paying attention!

IMAGINE YOUR HEART HAS EARS AND EYES

David Bohm, a very famous quantum physicist and colleague of Albert Einstein, once said, "When you listen to somebody else, whether you like it or not, what they say becomes a part of you."

Within the universal field, as it is called in quantum physics, we create another field between us—and if we bring God's presence into that field, we can be, or are, taught the truth of all things.

As you listen, sit or stand with the person, be in your heart and focus completely on them. You may or may not look at them—some people feel better-heard when you make eye contact with them intermittently, and others prefer consistent eye contact. Do nothing else. Plan no reply speech. Do not rehearse what you want to say while you are waiting for the gap in the conversation. Do not judge what they are saying as it comes out of their mouths.

Try and quiet your own inner dialogue if it's negative, but be aware that there is a big difference between negative inner dialogue and intuition or inspiration! Intuition is the *inner tuition* your heart's wisdom shares—it may be a knowing or a feeling about some action to be taken, or words to be said. Try to sense the difference.

When the person finishes speaking, slowly count to five before you say anything. Breathe in and out once before you speak. Respond to and acknowledge *how they feel*—not just their words—and be careful to respond and not to react.

You may say things like, "That must have been very frustrating for you" or "I imagine you were very disappointed when that happened." Other responses might be, "Wow. How did you manage to keep going? That must have been very hard" or "I am so sorry you felt I did that; that was not my intention." You could also say, "I am so sorry you perceived it that way and I can see how you could have" or "I can see your point of view and that it would have been very (insert feeling-based word here)."

It is a given that you are not sincere at this stage. This process is not part of what we normally learn about communication. If you are in your heart, you may not speak at all, but they will *feel* heard, deeply understood and safe. Don't be too concerned if you don't completely understand the content of what is being said. Listening involves more than comprehending what their *words* mean.

People generally are not interested in our opinions, thoughts or ideas—even if they ask! They are interested in feeling understood, validated and acknowledged. That is why our hearts need to have ears and eyes for feelings.

IT'S ABOUT THEM, NOT YOU

You will begin to understand now that communication is not about "us," it is about relating on a soul level. Miscommunication is rampant because many times what comes out of most people's mouths may not be what they really mean or feel.

Our hearts need to listen and sometimes internally reframe what a person is saying into what they really need or want, and then we respond to that out loud.

Sometimes it is difficult to truly listen, especially when the speaker is highly emotional. If this emotion is directed at us, we may feel defensive, judged or criticized. Remember that people's language usually communicates more about *themselves* than about you, no matter how it sounds or how you perceive it!

When we are only *hearing words*, we can become defensive—and perceive that we are being judged, criticized or attacked—whether we are or not. But if we remain in our hearts, trying to understand what a person is really *feeling*, we will be less likely to be trapped at the surface of words or emotional states. When you are good at heart-listening, what you say will make the other person feel truly understood!

Interrupting someone midsentence or midthought is not listening. When we interrupt, we have stopped listening and have been rehearsing our defensive or emotional volley of words. We can't even *wait* for the gap in the conversation before we react to the message we *think* we heard.

When we are operating as if *everything* that is said or done is about us and are not considering the soul level or that most communication is about the communicator, we can miss the point completely. We end up fearful, unhappy, angry, defensive and hostile about being attacked. The speaker feels totally unheard, dissatisfied, frustrated and disappointed. The issue remains unresolved and the atmosphere tense.

Remember, listening is about them—not about you.

SPEAKING

A section on listening needs a section on speaking. You will probably find you speak much less with *this* way of listening; however, speaking is part of the connection of communicating. Before you speak, think quickly and ask yourself, "Will this response be helpful to this person?" If your reply is no then wait a moment, and if nothing comes, respond in some appropriate way. Long awkward pauses can make conversations uncomfortable and difficult.

Choosing the right words is critical, but choosing the right way and time to say those words is more critical. If we only spoke goodness and gratitude, if we focused on the good about another, or in all situations, and that's all we let come out of our mouths or in our actions, we would be good connectors.

Imagine you are listening to God when you listen to others. It's a brilliant way to immediately transform communication. You wouldn't dream of speaking to God or some divine presence in a surly, defensive, belligerent, angry, critical, nasty, rude or derisive tone, with abusive words! Nor would you dream of listening to God with a mind full of judgment, ridicule and disgust, or of not listening with your total, undivided attention when He "speaks" to you!

As the spark of the Divine lives in all of us, then it would be wise to listen to and speak to that part of God or the Divine in everyone. In other words, from today onward, remember, every conversation you have is with God, no matter to whom you are speaking. Period.

DAILY SCHEDULE
SUNDAY: LISTEN TO GOD

"Listening is a creative force that transforms relationships. Listening is a sacred art. It is an awareness that not only are we present to each other, we are present to something that is spiritual, holy, sacred."[1]

—Kay Lindahl

God "talks" to us in many "languages." He also uses the body through gut feelings, instincts, intuition, inspiration, angels who appear in our lives as people or in dreams, a sense of knowing, books we read, advertisements we see, evangelists or speakers we watch, children, life dramas, misfortunes and more. He has to be this flexible because few of us ever stop to listen directly to Him!

I remember going to church one day, about a year after I had moved to Dallas from Australia. The pastor at Highland Park United Methodist Church, Mark Craig, had given another brilliant sermon. And I was once again crying! I didn't understand why this happened every time I went to this church. I would be perfectly okay before I went in, and within minutes, I would start to cry.

It was a different sort of crying from the usual. Tears would stream out of my eyes, but I wasn't crying like I do if I am upset. I started to think there was something wrong with me! That perhaps I was much more lonely than I thought. (Do you know that I just mistyped, "I was much more *lovely* than I thought." Was it a slip—or was God talking to me just then? Ha ha!)

After a while, I realized that many times when I went into that church, a feeling of love overwhelmed me. And I didn't know anyone in this congregation, and they did not seem particularly welcoming. It dawned on me that this was God's love I was feeling and I was crying with joy. (Duh. It takes some of us longer than others!)

Once I realized that, I felt more sane. I was also told recently that the Holy Spirit can move people to laughter, dancing or tears—cleansing tears—but that experience was a first for me.

But back to the day I was talking about. This particular day, I was sobbing, not just crying. I cried all the way home and thought, "What is wrong with me?" I wondered if I should read the Bible when I arrived home to see if there were any clues in it, because I had no idea what was wrong! (This was pretty unusual, as I did not read the Bible much then either.)

Once home, I could not read, as the tears were blurring my vision so badly. So I just had to sit there. (God was moving in his mysterious ways!) As I sat, I became aware of a feeling of being overwhelmed. I knew I had some big task to do, but I didn't know what it was, and I was sure I was inadequate for it, whatever it was!

After waking up to that, it was as if there was a guardian angel or some sense of a being, sitting and smiling benignly at me. I could not see or hear it, but I could sense it. I could sense the smile, and the love that was like that of an indulgent and patient parent, and I "heard" (but really sensed), "Do you think God would give you a task to do and not give you all the skills or the help you needed to do it?"

That was it. I stopped crying instantly. I smiled and thought, "Of course not!" I continued with my day feeling energized!

Have you ever had an experience with a similar result? I bet God tries to touch us all the time, and we don't stop long enough to hear Him unless we are facing a crisis.

Take time to pray and to listen to God. Ask Him what he wants you to do. What is His will for you? Are you on the right path? Importantly, ask Him how you can be a blessing to others. Ask Him to help you—and pray with joyful expectation. God hears every prayer and sends blessings and grace—so stay open and watch for the miracles. Be patient with a heart full of hope that the answer will come when the timing is perfect—for you—even though it might not look like it right now.

Always have the intention in your heart to be doing what God wants of you. Ask, "What do you need, God? What can I do for you today?"

Pray all the time, but part of prayer is "listening" to the answers He sends you. They may be in things you see or pass by, strangers you meet, your friends or family—you never know where the answer will

THE GOSPEL OF JOY

come from, so stay awake, be conscious and expect to find the answer somewhere.

He always answers. Always.

MONDAY: LISTEN WITH YOUR HEART FOR FEELINGS AND LET PEOPLE FEEL SAFE WITH YOU

When listening, accept people for who they are and try to "step into their shoes."

A great question to ask yourself when listening to another person is, "What does this person really need from me right now?"

Let your heart surround them and quiet your inner dialogue or thoughts. This helps you to be "in their shoes" and more accurately sense their feelings. Remember to see the *words* as *feeling wrappers*. Unwrap and reveal the essence of what they are speaking about—even if *they* are not conscious of it!

When you are this present with someone, sincerely desiring to understand, they feel secure, safe, loved, heard at a soul level, known for who they truly are, fully accepted and understood!

Think of your best friend—the one who knows you better than anyone and still loves you. They understand your little idiosyncrasies and annoying habits and still seek your company! They give you, and you give them, a safe space to be, and that allows interaction without fear of judgment, hidden agendas or confrontation.

Try and listen to everyone as if he or she were your best friend.

When you are on the phone, *stop and do nothing else* as you speak to your caller! In fact, close your eyes so you can tune in to them and the sound of their voice if that helps you. People can sense whether you are being attentive, even if you are not in the same location.

I know we live in a fast-paced and noisy world, but it is still important to give the speaker your undivided attention. Sit in a comfortable chair and listen as if they were sitting across from you. Cellular or cordless phones make this much more difficult, as we are inevitably doing other things while talking! We need the discipline to stop for important conversations and listen to people's hearts.

On the phone, we don't have the advantage of body language to help us work out what feelings are present. Although we can only use voice tones and breathing patterns to help guide us, our spirits know no boundaries. We can still listen and respond to them using the heart's wisdom. It may be a little more challenging, but with practice, we are able to listen deeply even over the phone.

What about those situations when you don't have time to truly listen or be present—to be in your heart and listen from there? I have found that people don't mind if I tell the truth. I say, "I am really sorry, but I am so busy right now that I cannot give you my full attention. Could we have this conversation in 20 minutes?" I always try to give a time frame and honor my commitment with that time.

If you are the one needing to talk with someone, and your prospective listener asks if they can have a little time to prepare themselves, understand and appreciate that this person genuinely does want to listen with their heart but cannot do it at this minute. You will appreciate their honesty and the undivided attention you receive when the conversation does take place.

Your mission today: To truly connect with others, and have your heart present with theirs; to do nothing else while you listen; and to make everyone you listen to feel safe by listening from your heart, accepting them and responding to the feelings wrapped in words. Then notice the difference in *your* life and *their* joy!

TUESDAY: WHY AM I BATTERING MYSELF?

We would never speak to our worst enemy the way we speak to ourselves!

Today may be a day of revelation. Have you ever spent a day consciously listening to how you speak to yourself?

Often, we say dreadful things to ourselves that we would never say to our friends—or even our enemies! We call ourselves idiots and think we are ridiculous. We judge ourselves constantly.

Some of us "should" ourselves a lot. We say things like "I *should* have done that better" or "I *should* have known that." And there is always the

"I am so embarrassed; I am so fat; I am such a loser; I suck at relationships." I could go on for pages and so could you, probably!

Who needs enemies when we treat ourselves like this!

This is the day you start treating yourself kindly and looking at yourself from your heart's perspective.

Step 1 is to become conscious of everything you say to yourself. Track it all day. Stop as soon as you become aware of something negative you said to or about yourself. Jot down the most common nasty phrases you use on yourself. Writing them down is important, as they look even more sinister (or silly!) on paper. And you can actually *see the phrases you are constantly repeating to yourself.*

Be on the alert, since many of us have a nasty inner voice—I call it the "criticizer"—that hangs over our heads and blocks us from receiving inspirations and truthful insights about ourselves. It appears faster than we can imagine, and before we know it, it has stopped any true listening and triggered a defensive reaction of anger, shame or one of a hundred troubling emotions that emerge because the criticizer has taken over.

The purpose of today is to become conscious of this self-destructive language. Repetition reinforces belief, so imagine the impact of telling yourself thousands of times how useless you are or what a loser you are or any of those other phrases you have written down.

Look at the list you have made of the criticizer's favorite lines—and make time today to question if they are:

1) True

2) Useful

3) Judgmental

4) Phrases that your father/mother/siblings/teachers/partners/ friends said to you years ago that stuck in your mind

5) "Stuff" that you took on and made your own even if it was not true or helpful

6) Observations that were true at one time but are no longer

This is a fabulous exercise to do with your children—no matter what age. Make sure they feel emotionally safe as you listen and help them. It will be one of the greatest gifts you can give them.

If you make the commitment to change, here is a simple and great technique. Find a rubber band large enough to be very loose around your wrist. (We want to keep your circulation going!) Those bands do not have any snap to them! They are stiff. To help you silence the criticizer, when you hear that voice or phrase, pull the rubber band far enough out from your wrist so that when it snaps back it stings slightly. Do not pull it out so far that it snaps back, hurts you or draws blood. Be responsible, sensible and kind to yourself—this is just a trigger to help you change your thought patterns!

Years ago, a researcher named Pavlov fed dogs and rang a bell each time he did. Within a short time, the dogs would salivate at the sound of the bell even if no food were present. Our old brains learn in this way—so the rubber band is just a fun and effective way to reprogram the mind. It will not make you salivate, but it really helps to stop negative thoughts or worry!

WEDNESDAY: LISTEN TO YOUR HEART

"As a man thinketh in his heart, so is he."

—Jesus Christ

The heart's wisdom is much gentler and quieter than our judgments. The pure heart is not judgmental, it is discerning. Some people choose to hate, trick, steal from or harm people—they do not have a pure heart. The voice of their conscience becomes fainter and they justify to themselves that it is okay to live this way. That's why discernment is so important.

Thoughts from a *pure* heart are true, wise and safe. The treasure a pure heart seeks is connection to God and working for the highest good of all. In the Sermon on the Mount, Christ said, "For where your treasure is, there will your heart be also." Is your treasure God and His ways or false gods such as possessions, control or power? Which do you long for? It will affect the choices your heart makes, your health and your destiny. You can discern what a person treasures by observing their behaviors.

Today is your day to "listen to" the pure heart's quiet voice. Compare the "voices" of your judgments with those of a pure heart. Which is louder and more insistent? Think about which one rules your behavior. Most of us are not conscious of the "competition" inside the heart, the choice between conscience and judgments. Judgment often wins because it's a more familiar pattern.

Most of us don't even know our heart has a voice—we only occasionally notice "gut feelings" or "intuition" or "we just have a sense" or, best of all, we just *KNOW* something is true or right or what we need to do. These are some of the ways the heart "talks" to you.

Our hearts create an electric current that is 60 times more powerful than any other organ in the body. The heart field is measurable and can affect another person's brain waves!

There is a doughnut-like electromagnetic field that emanates from the heart and connects us with all living beings. When the heart is pure and full of appreciation and gratitude, we change both its waves *AND* other people's. It is so much more than a pump! (Visit www.heartmath. com to learn more about the incredible power of the heart.)

For some people, listening to the heart is more easily done in silence. Initially you may need to find a quiet spot, but with practice you can tap into the heart's wisdom anywhere, because it's an awareness, a feeling and a state of being.

In this quiet spot, ask God to help. Quiet all the mental chatter to clearly hear the heart and be conscious of body sensations, inspirations, gut feelings or a sense that something is not right or as it should be. Clear hearts know what is best for us—we just have to learn the language.

To be awake to that knowing or the way the heart communicates takes a conscious effort. So we need to sit quietly and reflect for a few minutes. Invite the heart to speak. Ask your heart what you need to know. Be prepared for the answers to come in different ways. If the answers are judgmental or nasty, your heart's gentle whispering has been overridden. Start again!

If you feel peace when you have made a decision, it's probably your heart letting you know all is well. If you don't feel peace, better go back and double check!

See which makes you feel more peaceful, safer and happier, and feels more true, Judgment or heart speak!

It's a no-brainer!

THURSDAY: LISTEN WITH DISCERNMENT AND SPEAK ONLY GOOD

> "Everyone is God speaking. Why not be polite and listen to Him?"[2]
>
> —Hafiz

I love Hafiz's take on this. We all have that divine spark of God within us—and we *might* be God speaking sometimes or, more accurately, God might be speaking through us!

Many of us are polite but don't truly listen. Sometimes in our culture, being polite is merely pretense. I feel Hafiz meant be *present and kind* when he writes "polite."

It's time to go forth and see God in everyone—look for Him. Keep reminding yourself as you listen and speak that you are listening and speaking to God. Have the reverence that you would have for God for the people with whom you connect. Be aware of your voice tones, words, gestures, breathing and patience!

Today's challenge is also to speak only positive words. Not one negative word is to come out of your mouth or swirl around inside you. See the good in people and situations and say only good things about all others—and if you can't say anything good, say something neutral or don't say anything at all!

This will be an incredible day! God will be excited to be seen in so many places!

FRIDAY: ASK QUESTIONS

"I know that you believe you understand what you think I said, but I'm not sure you realize that what you heard is not what I meant."[3]

—Robert McCloskey

My wonderful Aunt Nancy was one of the real eccentrics in the world. She started life in India and had several husbands and maharajas in love with her as she lived an exotic life throughout several countries. I adored her!

She taught me many lessons—the most memorable of which was, "Darling, if you want someone to think you are interesting, listen to them, then ask questions about what they said. They will think *you* are fascinating!" She has been proved right time and again. People love being around someone who takes a sincere interest in them.

I am naturally curious and much prefer to ask questions—pertinent questions—than to speak. Everyone we meet *is* fascinating! They have rich stories and experiences, and most people so rarely listen and genuinely show interest that they think I am fascinating while I am busy finding *them* fascinating!

There is so much to learn in life, and most people love to share what they know. My husband is always in awe of what I find out about people, what they tell me, and how quickly I bond with them. I am sure it is largely in part because I *do* listen and I am genuinely interested. I am never certain what person God has chosen to give me a message, or through whom he will send help to me! It gives meeting everyone *and* anyone a whole new dimension.

Remember to ask questions that do not simply require yes or no answers all the time. Give people a chance to expand and share with you by asking questions that encourage them to give you more detail on what they have already told you.

Questions that begin with, "How did you. . .?"; "What was it that you found so . . .?"; "How specifically did the . . .?"; "When was the . . .?";

164

and "Can you expand on the bit about. . .?" are always conversation starters. Pay attention to the answers! If you are just asking questions to be polite, the person will know and you will *both* be bored!

Never be frightened of looking or sounding "stupid" because you ask a question. Be wary of judging yourself *before* you ask a question. I am never ashamed of not knowing something—none of us can know everything, and if I have not had an experience that has taught me about this subject, why would I judge myself badly? I just haven't had the opportunity to learn—until now—and I am grateful that this is my chance to find out! If you are interested, truthful and sensitive, and are being guided by the wisdom of your heart, asking a question is rarely offensive or insulting.

To start a conversation, ask questions like, "What's the best thing that happened to you today?" I love this one! Try it with your family every day—make it a ritual in the evenings over dinner—and watch the group dynamics change. It can be transformational when everyone knows you will ask them that question every night. They come home thinking about the answer because they know you will ask it! This is a small change with a monumental effect. Try it at staff meetings and see how the energy and vitality of meetings improves. You can even use it on your voice mail!

It's also important to share yourself, as well, because conversations are not a one-way street! And if someone seems interested in listening to you and your story, be willing to share it! (Hopefully this book will help create many listening experts!)

Michael Grinder (www.michaelgrinder.com) is another one of my mentors on communication. He is a master of nonverbal communication and an educator's educator. It is magical to see Michael in action with teachers and corporate groups, helping them become excellent communicators. I have studied with him for 15 years and wanted to share with you one of his strategies (with his permission) for helping improve our true listening skills.

When someone is speaking and they finish, WAIT. DO NOT SPEAK. (As Michael recently elaborated on this, he says "WAIT" really should stand for, "Why am I talking?) Instead of speaking immediately, nod, look down and reflect on what the speaker said. (I would describe this as unwrapping the feelings in that time.) Then count to five and if they say nothing more, THEN you can reply.

It is extraordinary how much more information someone will give you in that short space of silence. So few people give others even five seconds to add more, because they have been rehearsing their reply speech ever since the other person started speaking. Most of us are poised and ready to leap into the gap at the end of their sentence. We've already formulated our answer (instead of listening to what they said) and have been waiting impatiently for them to shut up so we can talk!

So ask questions, be interested in the answers, and when the speaker finishes, wait five seconds at least, unwrap the feelings and then—only then—talk! Persevere—it sounds easier than it is, but it's worth it!

SATURDAY: DISGUISES THAT WORDS TAKE ON

When you sense something is wrong and you ask, "What's wrong?" the word NOTHING takes on a whole new meaning!

I have learned so many lessons since I got married! I was 49 and my husband, 54. I had been single for about 20 years, and I thought I was Miss Communication Guru, but marriage has been a humbling experience. I really found out how little I knew! And that I was the *Miscommunication Guru!*

It has taken us two years to learn that what we say is not necessarily what we mean or need! My husband and I have had a number of "discussions" where there *appears* to be some specific issue with the cooking, car, house, garden or some tangible physical thing, when really it has nothing to do with those. They are just the words wrapping the feelings! How long it took me to recognize that!

It is incredible how the need to be acknowledged and to feel safe, loved and understood are at the bottom of so many silly little things we discuss. Okay, I really mean fights! (See how we use words to disguise things?) Feelings of insecurity, inadequacy or fear appear as arguments about who is going to navigate or do the shopping. Am I the only one, or have you noticed this in your relationships as well?

I am in awe of how I can be so unaware of my own feelings at times. For example, I wonder why I am making such a big fuss over money sometimes, when really I am needing to be validated for who I am!

The amygdala is part of the old brain and is the source of many of our deep, hidden fears. Our memories of emotional events are stored there, and years later, those feelings can surface under very different conditions from those in which they were created.

Under stress, the amygdala, which is *very* basic and acts as if it is responsible for our survival, takes over. Out of what seems to be no-where comes a disproportionate amount of fear, anxiety or anger for our current situation.

This is a *very* basic description of a very complex process so allow me poetic license. What I'm trying to do is highlight how often we don't even know the source of our weird reactions. We don't know that what we appear to be upset about has nothing to do with how we feel or what we really need!

So today is the day to notice the "disguises" words give to feelings. When a teenager says "I hate you"—do they really mean it? Or if they say they "hate school," is that the truth? Rarely. Most of the time they are scared about something, and our job is to find that fear and reassure them, or help them face it. Listen very, very carefully to teenagers—they bring great gifts with their "difficult" years! Apart from giving us "stress wrinkles," they can teach us to be experts at unwrapping feelings!

When people make judgments about others, it is often a projection of how they see themselves. If they are jealous, perhaps they are really telling themselves nasty things about how unattractive they are and comparing themselves with others. (For more help in this area visit www.thework.com. It is Bryon Katie's website and her techniques are very useful for helping us see how we cause a lot of our own pain with misperceptions, thoughts and beliefs!)

If we can wake up to our responsibilities and be conscious that the emotions of disappointment, anger and frustration are caused by *our* thoughts, then we can help both ourselves and others find joy.

Sometimes, trying to imagine what another person is thinking as they are speaking helps you respond more appropriately. Try also to sense if you need to back off and allow them some privacy. Timing is important! Or even asking the question, "What thought is causing you to feel this way?" may improve the other person's insight. Perhaps ask them, "What are you saying to yourself about this?" Then again, this may just make them angry! It really has to be done with great love, from your heart and with a sincere desire to truly listen and understand, at the right time.

Our voice tones need to be gentle when we ask these sorts of questions. The language must be the language of the heart, which reassures the person and allows them to feel safe. Remember to be wary of taking the meaning of any words literally—especially at times of stress. You will miss the real message being transmitted to you.

Deep listening is a hug you give the other person with your heart!

CHAPTER 9

A WEEK OF LAUGHTER

YOUR SEVEN MINUTES

Think of the last time you laughed so hard tears ran down your cheeks. Can you even remember it? Was it years ago?

Can you remember the last time you just laughed a lot?

What is the happiest time you can recall? Did you laugh a lot then? What made you laugh?

What usually makes you laugh? When you laugh, how do you feel? Where do you feel it?

When you hear little children laughing, how does it make you feel, and do you find yourself smiling or laughing as well?

Do you laugh enough?

How can you bring more laughter into your life?

AMANDA'S TAKE ON LAUGHTER

"What is laughter? What is laughter?
It is God waking up! O it is God waking up!
It is the sun poking its sweet head out

From behind a cloud
You have been carrying too long
Veiling your eyes and heart.

Oh, what is laughter, Hafiz?
What is this precious love and laughter
Budding in our hearts?

It is the glorious sound
Of a soul waking up!"[1]

—Hafiz

The poem above is a condensed version, and I encourage you to buy the book by Daniel Ladinsky and read all of Hafiz's poetry—your heart will be singing at the end of every page! Ladinnsky has translated and interpreted the wonderful writings of Hafiz, one of the best-known Sufi poets from Persia. The book is so joyful that laughter almost bubbles out of it just as it lies on my desk! And it certainly makes me feel good and touches my heart when I read it.

I really believe laughter *is* the sound of a soul waking up. Listen to a little child laughing hysterically and you will know that it's true! It *is* the sound of the soul stirring. It bubbles out from our hearts. How *alive* do you feel after a great laugh?

During my presentations, I use a lot of humor, although I never really designed it that way. Initially, I worked at making my presentations entertaining because I didn't want people to be in a coma at the end of an hour! But after 23 years, I am pretty much myself on stage, and what I speak about is so loaded with life humor that we all just laugh! I have fun, the audience has fun, and all our souls are happy and connected.

It is the most amazing transformation to see 7,000 (or 70) people light up and connect with laughter. They have just rushed in from stressful, busy lives burdened by problems and dramas and are overwhelmed with all they have to do. They are intense and focused and have furrowed brows. Most are disconnected from themselves and others, talking fast and unable to really "see" others.

But at the end of an hour of laughter, they're glowing. They have their arms around each other and their faces have relaxed. Many have let go of things they have been hanging onto. They have changed their perspective and lightened up and actually *feel* better because they have experienced the power of their hearts and the endorphins racing through their bodies!

Endorphins are the body's natural happy drugs. They are very powerful hormones—more powerful at pain relief than morphine. They make us feel great—happy, peaceful, relaxed and joyful. We cannot synthetically manufacture anything as powerful as endorphins, but humans can do things to produce them anytime!

A simple way to release them is to put a big "silly" grin on our faces. Seriously! Just put a big smile on your face—you will be releasing lots of endorphins! Someone did this as a scientific experiment and it works! I am not kidding. When we do this—fake a grin—I know you are not smiling and *you* know you are not really smiling, but our body-mind doesn't!

Instead, our body senses the muscles moving at either end of our mouths and our "crow's feet" muscles (for some of us!), which all send messages to the heart, digestive system and hypothalamus, which then tell the rest of our systems and soul to release endorphins.

So if you can't laugh, then at least put a big grin on your face, and you will soon start to feel better. And if you can't make it a huge grin, then just make a small smile and work your way up. (You may have to keep grinning for a while!) And if that doesn't work, then put a chopstick between your teeth and move your lips off it into a *huge* "grin." The chopstick technique does make you dribble a bit—but you release endorphins!

LAUGHTER AND HEALING

We *know* that laughter helps healing. Norman Cousins, in his book *Anatomy of an Illness,* was the first person to really write about how he healed himself from a fatal illness by checking out of hospital and working with laughter and optimism as his primary method of healing.

Laughter therapy is now an accepted and valuable form of treatment in hospitals and hospices.

Cousins writes that "laughter is a form of internal jogging. It moves your internal organs around. It enhances respiration." And it does! So it helps you breathe better and jiggles things around inside that need to be jiggled, which improves circulation, and then it gives you an endorphin high!

This is not a very scientific way to describe the studies that have actually been done on the health benefits of laughter, but they are very impressive. They are so significant that if you really want to help someone heal more quickly, help them laugh a lot. Keep everyone laughing around them to keep their spirits high. Even if you can make them smile, it will help and they will feel better because endorphins are reducing their pain.

We all need to laugh more, but our busy lives are not geared to encourage laughter. Children laugh about 300 times a day. Guess how often we grouchy old adults laugh? Seventeen. We need to improve this!

Laughter will help us keep our heart healthy, lower the stress hormones pumping around the body, boost the immune system, keep us younger and help us fight off disease and live longer.

Be vigilant: Consciously *create* opportunities to laugh. Watch comedy videos, movies or programs—not dramatic violence or news! Do you know that for about five hours after you watch a violent movie, your immune system is less robust, whereas comedy videos boost the strength of the immune system through laughter?

Laughter can even make you fitter! One study has shown that if we laugh 100 times in a day, it is the equivalent of rowing 10 minutes on a rowing machine or spending 15 minutes on an exercise bike. For me, laughing 100 times a day is WAY more fun than spending 15 minutes on an exercise bike!

FUNNY GLASSES

We need to develop a sense of humor that is creative and ever present. Look for funny things around you each day; they are everywhere. They could be funny street signs, babies laughing or animals being cute.

Once you set the intention to notice funny events and happenings, you will be surprised at how they "suddenly" appear everywhere! They have been there all along but you haven't noticed them before.

Here's an idea: Make yourself a set of "funny" glasses. Not funny-looking necessarily, but ones that magically make everything you see through them seem funny. (You have to pretend—be creative. They are a symbol, remember!) Wear them for a while each day so that when you have them on, the whole world is colored with "funny"! (These should be a reminder for us to consciously work at seeing humor, fun and joy in everything.) I know it's silly, but try it before you judge it. They might be very useful at work!

To teach children optimism, what fun it would be to have rituals in the home to consciously create humor! What if once a week, everyone in the family sat at the table and took turns at wearing the funny glasses while they talked about the funniest thing they saw, heard or thought that day. Or what if they talked about some difficult thing that had happened and tried to see the funny side of it?

Imagine the wonderful lessons you would be teaching children— and grown-ups—if this were part of a family tradition.

FUN FAIRIES

When I speak about the importance of laughter with groups, there are always a sad few who say, "Gimme something to laugh about!"

The problem is that there is no fun fairy who flits around, sees us being miserable and then changes everything by waving a magic wand over us!

We have to be our own fun fairies. We need to be the ones who bring ourselves joy and laughter. It seems that many people aspire to be a CEO, CIO, CTO, CSO or C-something in the corporate world, so as of today, you can become your own official CFF—*Chief Fun Fairy*.

This is your mission: Go forth and laugh 100 times or more every day and help others to laugh that often as well. (Well, at least laugh *more* than 17 times a day!)

In our office, we try to help people in their mission to be fun fairies by manufacturing magic wands that light up and make a *brrriiinngg* noise (they are available on our website, and you will hear the noise as soon as the first page opens up on www.amandagore.com).

They are very popular and work to make teenagers disappear, partners laugh, misery evaporate and all manner of other fun things! Use one at work to create magic but watch it carefully—everyone will want to use it! You can go further and buy some wings or even a fairy outfit, or just sprinkle fairy dust about. Who knows—you may have the best day of your life!

LAUGHTER—THE GREAT CONNECTOR

Comedian and musician Victor Borge said, "Laughter is the shortest distance between people."

I say *laughter is the great connector!* It connects individuals and groups, whether they are strangers or friends. Laughter overcomes arguments and difficulties, helps us lighten up and stops us from being so intense.

I feel God connects with people through laughter and He connects us to each other in the same way. Laughing *with* someone because you consciously try to see the funny side of the "drama" in which you find yourselves can transform everything. Laughter is an alchemical process as well—it can transmute pain and negative emotions into joy. Laughing *at* someone is unkind and *causes* pain.

Think of the most popular people you know; most of them are the "life and soul of the party." What does that mean? It means they are great connectors. They have the ability to entertain and to tell stories, and to help us laugh and make us feel better.

So many women tell me the thing they love most about their partners is that "he makes me laugh—even after all these years!" The ability to make someone laugh is a blessing and keeps us connected—we can all do it!

Dale Irvin, a wonderful speaker and friend of mine, has the most infectious laugh I have ever heard. I saw him recently and suggested he make a CD of his laugh so we can all have it handy and play it on the way to work, home or appointments to put us in a great frame of mind.

Do you have a friend with an infectious laugh who would not mind your taping it? Have a group of friends over one night for a laughter party—and tape the results! Or tickle and play with your toddlers and tape their precious laughter. (Now *that* recording would fill your heart, lift your spirit and make you laugh!)

All in all, laughter is wonderful for your heart and soul and great for your body. It connects you with others, puts things in perspective, releases "stuck stuff," heals and works—even if you fake it!

God blessed us with the capacity to laugh, so we should exercise that gift. God is playful. We need to be as well!

Voltaire said, "God is a comedian playing to an audience too afraid to laugh." Why let fear destroy one of the most precious gifts you have? Be brave! If you look silly, who cares? God and your body love it when you laugh.

DAILY SCHEDULE

SUNDAY: SMILE AND STOP TAKING YOURSELF SO SERIOUSLY

"Everyone smiles in the same language."

—Anonymous

Today, your task is to smile all day. Smile at everyone. Greet complete strangers with a smile and you'll notice that most of them smile back. Smile at little children (we tend to do that automatically anyway). Smile at your neighbors even if you don't like them!

Smiling uses far fewer muscles than frowning, and if I am going to have wrinkles (I should actually say MORE wrinkles!), then I would rather have laughter lines than frown lines! Remember, smiling releases endorphins, so no matter how bad you feel, it's a powerful way to change the physiological makeup of your body.

Smiling is the doorway to lightening up!

When I arrived in the U.S., I had no idea there would be a cultural gap. I figured we all spoke English and watched the same television programs and were very similar. WRONG! There is a cultural chasm—not a gap—between Australia and America!

The best way I can describe that chasm is in how seriously we take ourselves—or not! If you think you are very important and take yourself seriously in Australia, it is amazing how quickly someone comes up and lets you know just how insignificant you really are!

Really! It's a cultural phenomenon called the "tall poppy syndrome," where someone who stands out from the pack is cut down so we are all equal. It may be harsh but it does make Aussies very difficult to offend! And we sure don't take ourselves too seriously. We find it easy to laugh at ourselves, and when we do, life is lighter!

My audience laughs a lot when I mention how many Americans seem to be intense! (Not those of you reading this, of course!) Some people take themselves *soooo* seriously. In Australia, we have a phrase for people like that: "They are so far up themselves, it's dark!"

Today is the day to smile *and* laugh at yourself! Catch yourself if you are taking yourself and life too seriously. Work toward lightening up and loosening up. Let go of who you are supposed to be or what position you are in, and be playful.

It is absolutely possible to be professional *and* have fun. Just because you are an accountant, a lawyer or a medical professional, for example, doesn't mean you can't have fun while you work!

In fact, people love to think that they can go to their accountant's office to talk about serious financial matters and still have a laugh and feel good when they leave. It's my belief that if you are truly professional at what you do, you will take your work seriously but not yourself.

I took my work as a physical therapist extremely seriously—and yet we all did silly things and had a great time. I also take my speaking very seriously, but if you saw me onstage, you would know that it looks nothing like serious. But the message and the way I impart it are very carefully crafted and wrapped in great laughter to create the maximum benefit for the audience members. So if you are a "professional," this is your day to make your interactions fun while taking the work seriously!

I read a magazine story some time ago about a man at an airport. As often happens in the u.s., weather had caused the cancellation of a lot of flights. There were long lines at the ticket counters. This man stormed up to the desk, pushing in front of a long line of people, banged his hand down on the desk and shouted, "I need to fly to Chicago!"

The airline person said as kindly as she could, "I am sorry, sir, and I will help you as quickly as I can. If you could just stand in line." He looked at her, slammed his hand down again and said, "Do you know who I am?"

She stopped, motioned for him to wait, picked up her microphone and announced over the loudspeaker, "Ladies and gentlemen, there is a man at Counter 23 who does not know who he is. If anyone does know who he is, could they please come forward?"

What a great story!

Slow down and realize that the world does not revolve around you. Stop being offended! Most people are not out to "offend" us on purpose—in fact, no one can "offend" us. We take offense! We interpret what they say, make judgments about what they do, make assumptions about their intentions, and then we talk ourselves into being offended!

Do you ever wake up and think, "I want to offend someone today?" Most people don't! Save yourself a lot of pain and give people the benefit of the doubt, or at least see the humor in situations instead of taking offense.

Smile—even if you don't feel like it! Lighten up. Laugh. Wake up your soul!

MONDAY: REMEMBER ALL THE FUNNY TIMES IN YOUR LIFE

"Laughter is very powerful medicine. It can lower stress, dissolve anger and unite families in their resolve to overcome troubled times."

—Anonymous

This should be a fun day. Plan to wake up ten minutes early and have a journal beside your bed. Spend those ten minutes recalling as many significant laughter-filled events in your life as you can. Write them down so you remember them all.

A favorite memory of mine happened one New Year's Eve. I can still picture the scene.

I was standing in the doorway between the kitchen and living room in my friend's house, insisting on reading aloud passages from Dave Barry's book *Dave Barry Turns 40*. This is a laugh-out-loud book, and I just *knew* everyone would love it. But as I was reading, I was laughing so hard that I had tears running down my face and I couldn't keep speaking! I was snorting with laughter!

By now, of course, the other guests had no idea what I was saying but they were laughing hysterically at me laughing! It was one of the best New Year's Eves I had ever had!

I didn't mind being the source of laughter—who cares if you look silly! I am the one doing the internal jogging and waking up my soul and sharing the gift!

When my nephew, Thomas, was a toddler, he used to run towards me with arms outstretched and face glowing with joy. Not only would I laugh, but my heart would burst with joy as he did this. Watching my beloved niece and nephew play, laugh and talk gave *me* endless hours of laughter and joy.

Combine all the video footage of your children laughing and playing so you have 20 or 30 minutes of unbridled joy that you can experience over and over again. This makes a wonderful gift for your children when they are older as well.

When my mum was in the hospital in the last weeks of her life, I arrived from the U.S. with a bag full of my little smiley-face finger puppets (I call them endorphins). They are bright yellow and have a smiley face on them and little arms stretching out either side. I put them all around her room. I tried to give them to the nurses and doctors, and do you know the really sad thing? Only one doctor and one nurse laughed and played with them. The others were not the least bit interested. Maybe they were asleep during the healing-and-laughter segment in their training!

Luckily, my brother Simon, who is one of the funniest people on earth, arrived, and the three of us had a hysterical time playing with those things.

If you have someone you love in the hospital, take as many fun things as you can in there and surround them. I had furry blobs that would endearingly laugh when thrown against a surface. I brought toys that sang songs, and funny hats and magic wands—anything that I thought I could use to help Mama and, as importantly, the medical staff, smile.

I wanted her surrounded with joy and laughter when I was not there. Some of my most precious memories of my mama are of that last week, and of her and Simon laughing. Mama had, and still has, I am sure, a great sense of humor, and she laughed often. She was always doing fun, silly things, and her children inherited that wonderful trait. It is a great blessing to be free enough to have fun without being worried about looking silly.

When I was a physical therapist, I used to have the most fun with my patients. We would laugh a lot even when I was encouraging them to do difficult, painful exercises; no matter how sick they were, I would help them laugh. I had not been taught to do that, but I instinctively knew how important it was for them to have fun. Clowning in hospitals is now an accepted form of therapy in children's wards—pity it isn't in the grown-up's ward, since we adults need to laugh more than children!

So today, recall and write down as many funny life moments as you can think of, and tomorrow you'll be making an album in which to keep those memories.

P.S. Make sure you discuss as many of these moments as you can at the dinner table tonight—it should mean you have a fabulous evening!

TUESDAY: **FIND PHOTOS OF AS MANY FUN TIMES AS YOU CAN**

"Laughter is the shock absorber that eases the blows of life."

—Anonymous

If you have children, I guarantee you have photos of them in your wallet. Not always to brag with, of course! But so that when you look at them, you feel your heart stir with joy.

Apart from the photos in your wallet, hopefully you have lots of other "magic laughter moment images" somewhere in your house or on your computer.

Today is the day to find them and put them in two or three small albums. Keep one at work, one at home, and carry one with you. Or if an album is too big, take one photo and laminate it. Look at it every time you want to laugh or smile.

Put several of your favorite pictures into photo frames—or make a collage of them in one frame. Place them on your desk and in prominent places at home. The photos we usually display are those in which we are perfectly groomed and carefully choreographed but they don't make us laugh! Instead, find the ones where you may not look so good, but anyone looking at that photo would not be able to avoid smiling and being touched by the joy jumping out of it.

If you scrapbook, imagine the fun you will have making a specific family-laughter album! As I sit here typing, I am surrounded by four photos of my mama, pictured with my brother and family in various stages of laugher. As therapy after she died, I made collages in large photo frames of laughter in her life. She brought joy to many people and I wanted to capture that for others. That way, I too remember her with laughter and gratitude and I stop focusing on my own pain—pain that doesn't help her!

Use your fun photos as screen savers on your computer. That works really well. Create a laughter album and make that a slide show as your screen saver. Imagine how good you will feel when you are taking a quick break if you see a series of joy-filled photos of you and your family or friends laughing. It will energize you for the rest of the day!

Digital cameras these days are small and easy to carry. Carry one with you everywhere so you can capture those unexpected laughter moments on film. They are treasures. They are moments of souls waking up and dancing. Every time you look at them, *your* soul does a little jig!

If you don't have any photos of your own, do an Internet search for funny pictures or funny video clips. The best video I ever saw (and I wish I could include it in the book!) was of a panda bear mother and her cub. The mother is sitting in the corner of a cage noisily chewing on some food. Her teeny little baby panda is lying at her feet sound asleep. Suddenly the teeny baby has a HUGE sneeze! And the mother nearly jumps out of her fur! It is the funniest thing to watch, and I keep it on my desktop and watch it every so often just to laugh!

Be creative about all the ways you can surround yourself with triggers for laughter. Maybe you and your family can sit at dinner together tonight and brainstorm ways to do it.

WEDNESDAY: WATCH A MOVIE THAT MAKES YOU LAUGH OUT LOUD

"A smile starts on the lips, a grin spreads to the eyes, a chuckle comes from the belly; but a good laugh bursts forth from the soul, overflows and bubbles all around."

—Carolyn Birmingham

There will be at least one movie in your life that has made you laugh out loud. Find that movie and watch it tonight if you can.

For me, it's *The Pink Panther Strikes Again*. No matter how many times I see it, I laugh. Silly Inspector Clouseau and his classic line, "Does your *durg* bite?" always makes me laugh out loud! (If you have not seen it, I highly recommend it!)

Other favorites are *There's a Girl in My Soup* and *Hitch*. Many people love the *I Love Lucy* series. Lucille Ball's facial expressions are hysterical!

Or the best funny movie of all—old family videos! Nothing makes you laugh more than watching you, your children or your family members from years before.

My sister had all our ancient baby movies that were on film transferred onto video. One of the funniest and most treasured nights of my life was sitting with watching them. We watched the same little segment about 20 times and were snorting with laughter! It was even funnier in reverse! (Being a little odd, I just love it when I am laughing so hard I snort! Not because I snort, but because it's a sign of how much laughing is going on!)

No one else would have laughed so hard watching this video because it was of me, about two years old, very chubby, in a funny little bikini doing nothing but jumping in and out of a wading pool, but Mama and I had a fabulous time. It was even funnier in reverse!

Vince and Michelle, the parents of our godchildren, have a hysterical video of the time Vince proposed! At the end of the "movie", the camera is filming the sky and ground because Michelle, who was holding the camera, was laughing so hard she couldn't keep Vince in the frame. It's all funny but that's the funniest part! Can you find something like that? Or create one?

If all else fails and you can't find a movie that's funny, what about taping or watching the television show *America's Funniest Home Videos?* (I have to admit that some of those seem brutal rather than funny.) Or make your own funniest home videos—plan a night where everyone in the family is in front of the camera doing funny things. This is also very good blackmail material to use with teenagers! (Just joking!)

If all that fails, play charades! That's almost like a movie and guaranteed to make you all laugh out loud!

There are many movies and roads to laughter. Your mission today is to find one for you and your family.

THURSDAY: LAUGH AND HELP OTHERS LAUGH

"Mirth is God's medicine. Everybody ought to bathe in it."

—Henry Ward Beecher

Today's mission is just to laugh out loud and to help others laugh. Laugh when you wake up, on the way to work, at work, in stores, on the way home, on public transport—wherever you are, laugh out loud at least once! Watch how others around you smile with you! It doesn't even have to be real—you can fake it and it still works!

One of the things I often have audiences do is to laugh hysterically. On demand!

When I introduce the idea, everyone groans, moans and grumbles. But then they start, and what begins as fake becomes genuine. All I can say is that watching a room full of thousands of people laughing out loud is alchemical!

Laughing changes the audience and the group dynamics, and often transforms the way they look at life and themselves. The only reason people grumble about the exercise is because they feel silly and are concerned about "what others will think"—which means they are frightened other people will judge them as silly! But God loves it when you laugh!

To help others laugh, it's important to laugh with them or at yourself but not at other people. This is obvious, but some people need reminding!

Laughing at other people shuts your soul down—and extinguishes their spirit. Helping others laugh can transform their perspective on the world. You can really make a difference in someone's life today just by helping them laugh at something.

If you are thinking, "I am not a funny person," you don't have to be! You can ask questions that elicit laughter from the person. Consider asking them about the funniest memory they have, or have them tell you stories about their children's most classic lines. No parent/aunt/uncle/godparent escapes without some fabulous little tales about toddlers who do something that is so funny you have to walk into another room and burst into laughter!

Or ask them about the funniest movie they have seen or funniest book they have read. You don't have to tell jokes or be the "life and soul of the party" to help others laugh!

Today you could also try spending time with the funniest people you know. There are always people you can talk to who make you laugh or with whom you laugh—call them on the phone and bring joy to their life today!

It doesn't matter what you do to create laughter today as long as it is respectful. Just laugh!

Children are always a wonderful source of laughter. This was one of those anonymous emails sent around the world. If you can't think of anything to help others laugh, read the following to as many people as you can. If you are the author, please let me know so I can acknowledge you!

JACK (age 3) was watching his mom breastfeeding his new baby sister. After a while, he asked, "Mom, why do you have two? Is one for hot and one for cold?"

MELANIE (age 5) asked her granny how old Granny was? Granny replied she was so old she didn't remember anymore. Melanie said, "If you don't remember, you must look in the back of your panties. Mine say 5 to 6." (I LOVED THIS ONE!)

JAMES (age 4) was listening to a Bible story. His dad read, "The man named Lot was warned to take his wife and flee the city but his wife looked back and was turned to salt." Concerned, James asked, "What happened to the flea?" (SO CUTE!)

And this one is a classic.

"Dear Lord," the minister began, with arms extended toward heaven and a rapturous look on his upturned face. "Without you, we are but dust." He would have continued, but at that moment, a 4-year-old girl leaned over to her mother and asked quite loudly, "Mom, what is butt dust?"

Go forth and laugh and make someone laugh today.

FRIDAY: MAKE A LAUGHTER JOURNAL AND READ FUNNY STUFF

"What soap is to the body, laughter is to the soul."

—Yiddish proverb

If you don't have any of Dave Barry's books, buy one them today. I think he is one of the funniest men on earth. I especially enjoyed *Dave Barry Turns 40,* but if you're under 40, perhaps another book would work for you.

Another book that I still love is the original A.A. Milne version of *Winnie the Pooh.* I remember when I was a little girl of about five, I would make Mum sit on my bed each night and read it over and over again. (You know how little children do that!) I loved the section on catching a "heffalump." I used to laugh and laugh and laugh and she would laugh and it was the most magical of times!

What a gift for your children to find a book they love to read that makes them laugh. Do you have any like that you can read to your children? You will both benefit. Sadly, our godchildren don't think the heffalump story is as funny as I did, but I still make them listen to it while I laugh! And then they laugh because I am laughing. So it still works! They think I am a dork, but I am quite proud of that!

Reading helps us develop, learn and grow, and if we can laugh as well, it's a major whammy! We learn, grow AND are filled with endorphins!

Have you read a book or story that makes you laugh out loud? Maybe you can compile all the funny stories that make you laugh into one document and create your own funny, laugh-out-loud book! What if you write your own funny material? Well, at least *you* would find it funny. Or keep a fun journal or laughter journal—write down things that happen to you every day or each week that made you laugh or that you found funny. Put photos in it or drawings of things you saw—be creative!

Imagine how much fun you would have reading that every few months. What if your family created a family fun album on which you worked once a week or more? I think that would be a fabulous activity for everyone and teach children wonderful lessons. (You might need your own adult version as well!)

Whatever material or book you find that makes you laugh, read it today and keep it handy. Commit yourself to reading more humorous books and finding funny books for your children. If cartoon books make you laugh, read those. I love reading Bill Cosby's books as well. His sense of humor is spectacular and appeals to almost everyone.

Whatever works for you—find some funny things to read or write. And laugh out loud! P.S. You might let people know your favorite authors so they can buy you books for birthday presents.

SATURDAY: TURN AROUND TOUGH MEMORIES WITH LAUGHTER

Laughter will transform memories.

This is going to sound a bit odd but it works!

If you can tell a story of something difficult in your life while keeping a smile on your face as you tell it, something magical happens to the chemicals linked with that memory. As we smile and tell the story, we might initially find it difficult. We need to ask the friend who is listening to remind us to keep smiling as we tell the story, and that often makes everyone laugh.(This works best with medium-sized memories, not the giant traumas of life.)

The most amazing things happen when we do this exercise. It is as if the body reprograms the memory and takes away some of the pain. Try it! I have done this many times and with others as well—and it really does work.

Look for the humor in difficult memories. This may take some work, but if you can find something funny about what happened or how you reacted, the pain of the memory diminishes or disappears. In your mind, scroll through events that still bring pain to your life and see if you can find some humor in them—especially embarrassing moments! They are always good for a laugh *with* yourself.

This is one of my most, if not *the* most, embarrassing memories:

When I was 21, I had finished college and was very naïve. I moved away from home into a house with four other people about my own age or a little older. They were doctors, teachers or lawyers and all appeared to me to be very sophisticated. They teased me mercilessly—especially about boyfriends—and often had many good laughs at my expense!

The worst trick they played on me was cruel. I had a crush on the psychiatrist in our little household, that says a lot about me just by itself.

He didn't know how I felt, but I believed the world was full of good and kind people, so I told the other female in the group, a teacher, of my crush. One day I came home from work and she and the lawyer rushed up to me and said, "John (the psychiatrist, name changed) wanted us to give you this." I unwrapped the cheapest, nastiest friendship ring I had ever seen! A normal adult at this stage would have laughed and seen right through the plot—but not naïve me!

The whole saga would take too long to tell, but I was worried about offending anyone and hopeful that John might have some interest, so I played right into my roommates' hands! This torture lasted for a few hours, with all members of the household playing along, weaving this yarn.

It took me about a week to laugh hysterically at the thought of what went on, but I still went bright red when I thought about it! Today I don't go red at all! The pain of embarrassment was transformed in my memory banks with that laughter.

Use this important technique on some of your present tough life situations. Search, dig and delve to find something funny about what is or was going on. In your mind, "stand outside" or "step back" from the situation and observe you, the situation or others. From this perspective, we can often see the funny side of things!

Remember, stuff happens and there is always some lesson for us to learn—even if it's just to lighten up and laugh at ourselves!

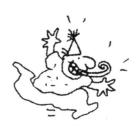

10

A WEEK OF LOVE

"Love is patient, love is kind. It does not envy, it does not boast, it is not proud. It is not rude, it is not self-seeking. It is not easily angered, it keeps no record of wrongs. Love does not delight in evil but rejoices with the truth. It always protects, always trusts, always hopes, always perseveres. Love never fails."

—I Corinthians 13:4-8

YOUR SEVEN MINUTES

When you think of love, what does it really mean to you? Do you just think of romantic love or family love?

Whom do you love? Who loves you? Who *unconditionally* loves you?

Would you call yourself a loving person? How do you behave when you are being loving? What gestures or words do you use?

Do you love yourself? Look deeply—do not answer this one lightly!

When you feel love for someone, where do you feel it in your body?

What feeds you with love? Can you recall a time in life when you "glowed" with light you were so loved? Or have you seen others glowing with the light of love?

How does someone look when they are loved? Or loving?

Find the different types of love in your life, and reflect on them.

AMANDA'S TAKE ON LOVE

Love is alchemical; it transmutes everything and saves the world. Joy is love laughing!

Most of us think immediately of romantic love when we see the word "love"—that stuff of intimate relationships. NO! *No, no, no, no, no, no!* Love is that but also *so* much more!

Love saves the world. The difference between "word" and "world" is the letter "L," which could stand for love, laughter, learning and listening. The flow of love is a force that can save the world. It holds the world together. It cushions us. It nurtures us. We *are* love. All of us.

Love is buried a bit deeper in some people—perhaps some type of shovel will work to find it in most cases, but sometimes a heavy-duty digging tool is needed to unearth that love!

In our hearts we can all access love. That is where we connect with God, the angels and the Divine, or whatever it is you believe in. Have you noticed that no matter what religion or belief system you explore, they all have love as the core or main philosophy?

Unfortunately, our lives, egos and personalities spin sheathes, membranes and fields around our heart, blocking the flow of love. Some people have never known love and don't know how to be loving—or loved.

Our task this week is to remove the veils so we can have access to, and love, our true selves; to open our hearts to God's love and give away as much love as we can. That is how more love comes into our lives. Beyond the veil, you will see the astonishing light you are. (You'll probably need dark glasses!)

Love comes in all sorts of shapes and sizes. It comes wrapped in gratitude, hope, kindness, laughter, joy, compassion, empathy, blessings, mercy, grace or play, or in just giving people your time. There are not enough pages to list all the way love manifests! Whenever you are engaged in those activities, you are feeling, receiving and giving love.

Love is poured out of the heavens into our hearts, and the more we give away, the more love pours in—it is a never-ending flow. Never hoard or keep love to yourself—it shrivels your heart and makes the divine stream dry up!

LOVE IS THE PLAYGROUND FOR SPIRITUAL GROWTH

The heart is the organ of love. It receives love from God and it fills us up. We glow and radiate it to others in our actions, thoughts and words. When we are full of real love, we are like a magnet to others!

If we listen to divine love and draw that into our hearts, we will always be guided truthfully. One of the ways we can love people is to fill our hearts with God's love and light and then shine that light on everyone we meet.

Have you seen those many religious paintings and icons that are of Christ or Mary or an angel, where their heart is lit up and often has a beam of light radiating forth? Imagine you are doing that with every person you meet. Try to see the rays as a gift from God to you and them.

I do this when I am speaking—I imagine a stream of golden white love light (a light filled with love as compared to plain old light!) coming from my heart and filling the room. I ask Christ beforehand to fill the room with His light and love, and then I "ray" out!

Try it before you scoff at it! You can do this with the person or people in front of you, or you can do it by imagining them in front of you and seeing or sensing the love light shining out over them.

Love is the playground for spiritual growth. We can practice, learn, stumble or laugh, and love picks us right up and dusts us off, just like we would if our learning-to-walk toddler had fallen for the hundredth time!

For me, God, Christ and love are the same thing. Love is everywhere. We just need to wake up, see it, feel it, tap into it and live in—and from—that flow. Once we are in the flow, we change.

Our job is to keep the stream of love flowing through us, and the world, by doing things that are filled with love for others.

HOW TO CONNECT TO LOVE, TRUE PRAYER AND GIVING

How do we connect with the love that is around us? Do everything you have read so far in this book! Be grateful. Talk with God from your heart. Pray. Listen to Him. Ask His forgiveness. Have joyful, hope-full expectations. Wait patiently with faith. Be compassionate. Do loving acts. Give love. Love yourself. Then you can be kind, judge not, see God in everyone you meet, use your heart as your guide, give, give and then give some more—there are so many ways!

God is always connected to us. We may not always feel connected to Him, but we have the capacity to become aware of that connection. Some forget that capacity or struggle with it at times.

Once we realize that the results of true prayer are powerful, we understand we should always begin with prayer. True praying means coming from deep within our hearts, with real faith, feeling, humility and reverence.

This is a selection from the New American Bible, in a letter from James 1:3-5:

> "For you know that testing of your faith produces perseverance. . . .
> But if any of you lacks wisdom, he should ask of God who gives to all generously and ungrudgingly and he will be given it. But he should ask in faith, not doubting. For the one who doubts is like a wave on the seas that is driven and tossed about by the wind. For that person must not suppose that he will receive anything from the Lord since he is a man of two minds, unstable in all his ways."

And again in Chapter 4, verse 3:

> "You do not possess because you do not ask. You ask but do not receive because you ask wrongly to spend it on your passions."

If your prayers seem unanswered, your faith may need to be stronger or you may be "double-minded," or what you were asking for was not the best thing for you, the world or another for whom you were praying. Praying for God's will in a situation is always wise!

Prayer takes practice, faith and consciousness. When we pray only for ourselves, our own pleasures or something we want, it does not work. When we request things that will be of benefit to others and us, and will help us in some way to do good or bring love into the world and make a positive change, God answers our prayers—in His own time! Any gift from God is a gift to you for others.

Many people think life is just about our own satisfaction or spiritual growth, but it's not. We are here to do things—to make this world a different place, to contribute what only we can do or think, whether it is to scrub floors, arrange flowers, paint or build skyscrapers.

Each person has to do what their heart leads them to do, and to love doing it. We don't all have the same gifts. Feel what gifts you have in your heart—feel what you are moved to do, what you have a passion for, what you love to do. Then ask God if you were right with what you felt! And ask for His blessing.

If we really want to connect with love, then we need to allow it to flow through us to others. This sounds simple and it is! It's not so easy sometimes, but it is simple.

If you did nothing else as a result of reading this chapter other than give more love and serve others, your life would change. Give in everything, but especially love and thanks.

Give away what you no longer use—or some of the things that are useful or mean a lot to you! Give to people who have less than you and more than you. Give of yourself, too. Be generous with your love; there is plenty to go around.

I believe I have prospered and grown in my business and life because I give all I can. Whatever I learn, I share. I don't hold anything back. (This drives some people nuts, of course, but it doesn't stop me from giving!)

If I can't give out loud, then I give in silence. I hold people in my heart if I am unable to give at an earthly level. Mind you, this kind of giving is probably the best I can do and I should start there. (See, I am learning as I type!)

I still have gazillions of lessons to learn, as we all do, but I strive to be mindful, and eventually, I catch myself when my spirit becomes mean. As soon as I am aware of it, I stop, and if I can't change how I feel, I put the people in my heart and hold them there and ask God to help me—and them.

Stop being frightened that if you give something up, there will be less for you. That's not a law! Life does not work that way. Your fears do.

Have faith and stay in the flow of giving and receiving love.

ROMANTIC LOVE

"There is an immense difference between love and desire."[1]

—Claire Blatchford

FALLING IN LOVE—WITH WHOM?

I have had many life lessons about romantic love, as have most of us. What have I learned? When we "fall" in love with another, we fall into seeing ourselves as we truly are. The other person initially sees us in all our glory, they reflect that to us, and we fall in love with our true selves—our "I AM"! We see what God sees in us.

We feel light, wonderful, joyful, loving and loved. Our spirit expands; we are more generous, giving and gracious with everyone. We look fabulous and our eyes sparkle. (Have you ever noticed how people who are in love have eyes that sparkle?) Everyone knows that something great has happened to us.

At some stage, this special person sees our warts. And *we* see our warts. And then our newly found self-love falters. We remember all the bad stuff, and instead of seeing ourselves as God sees us, we allow the criticizer back in! And then we fall out of love.

We do the same for our partners, by the way! They fall in love with us because through us, they fall in love with their true selves. If only we could live with the image of ourselves as they first saw us—that is the real us anyway! Can you remember how lovable you were and how wonderful you felt when you fell in love?

If we can learn to love ourselves, warts and all, as God does, we become love "radiators." Then we can accept and love someone *else*, warts and all as well! (And remember, warts can be contagious!)

OUR SPIRITUAL TEACHERS

"For one human being to love another: that is perhaps the most difficult of our tasks; the ultimate, the last test and proof, the work for which all other work is but preparation."

—Rainer Maria Rilke

The people with whom we have intimate relationships are a gift to help us grow spiritually. Everyone is our teacher, but we can grow more (and often more painfully) with those closest to us than with most others! These relationships and growth involve sacrifice, which is one of the cornerstones of love.

Think about it—what is compromise? We sacrifice our selfish wants or ego for another. We are always looking out for them, trying to see things as they see them and being there for them. We serve them. Intimate relationships offer us a great opportunity to become less selfish.

So the next time you are in the middle of a huge argument and you are ready to scream at your partner, stop, and in a state of awe and wonder, look at them in a new light. Look at them as a spiritual teacher! Feel incredibly grateful that they are putting themselves through all this pain so you can learn! Then look at yourself to find the lesson you are supposed to be learning. If nothing else, this little exercise takes the focus off the (most likely) trivial thing over which you are fighting!

Making the effort to grow together spiritually can lead to a love that is much deeper and more fulfilling than romantic love. It is calmer, gentler, more harmonious, safer, more profound and more satisfying, and it nurtures the real you. It takes work, but everything good takes work. Stick with it because it's worth the effort.

GREED AND SELFLESSNESS

If you want a steep lesson in learning how to grow out of selfishness, have children. One of the greatest sacrifices in my life has been *not* to have my own children. I have been blessed with nieces, nephews and godchildren I adore. I can't imagine loving my own children more, so I can feel, by proxy, some of the lessons a parent learns, but I have to rely on God to help me be selfless. He is still working on it!

If you are a parent, silently bless your child for the sometimes excruciating lessons they bring!

Whatever you do, do it with love. Strive to always have love as your motivating force or guiding intention. Make sure that love comes from your heart so it is pure. Unless we are very alert, we are easily fooled that we are doing something for someone because we love *them*, when really we have a selfish motive. Be aware of anything you do that is influenced by greed, manipulation, coveting, hate, revenge, anger or fear, and don't do it!

Greed and power separate; love connects. Greed and power constrict and weigh us down; love expands and lightens us. Greed and power harden; love soften. Greed brings more greed, and power brings a desire for more power; love brings peace. Greed and power bring suffering; love brings joy.

Make a sign for your home that says, "Have I given into greed today?" Talk to your children about greed, power and control, but also teach them about selfless love, sharing, valuing time together and non-materialistic qualities. These signs and discussions help us be conscious of what is motivating or driving us.

Stay awake and alert. Catch greed before it catches you and steals your capacity to love.

UNCONDITIONAL LOVE

As far as I know, God, Christ and Buddha could give unconditional love although very few humans ever have. Often our mothers or fathers, perhaps really, really good friends, and probably many of us, have had *moments* of unconditional love. Well, maybe!

People may love us *despite* our warts, they may love us *and* our warts, and some may truly unconditionally love us. And you are blessed if you have one person in your life who can do that.

Pure unconditional love is rare. It's a choice. We can *choose* to love and totally accept a person no matter what warts we see. As we unconditionally love and accept, we bring that capacity out in others.

I think truly loving someone (preferably everyone!) unconditionally is the lifelong journey for most of us. I can't even imagine how pure God's love is. It is always there and never wants anything but the best for us, and constantly forgives us. It pours grace and compassion over us, helps, accepts and supports us, and wants nothing back.

I feel love for my husband. I feel it for my family and friends, especially my mother. But honestly, I feel that I cannot love someone well enough to say I love them unconditionally, but I am working on it!

LOVE YOURSELF

> "You, yourself, as much as anybody in the entire universe, deserve your love and affection."
>
> —Buddha

Claire Blatchford has written a series of wonderful books (*Becoming: A Call to Love, Turnings* and *Friend of My Heart*) that are "must-haves" if you want to know about love.

Deaf from early childhood, Blatchford developed her inner listening capacity and discovered an "inner friend." The friend in her books is Christ. What He has told her in these books is just beautiful. Even if you don't believe in Christ, the books are worth reading.

Remember how, in the discussion of romantic love earlier, I said that falling in love with another is really falling in love with our true selves? And that the person who loves us sees us as the best we can be? Notice that I said, "can be." We can be like that! We are like that in our purity, in God's eyes. The difference is He can see our potential and is still loving and patient with us while we strive (or not!) to reach that potential!

Most of us have had at least one experience of being "in love," when every aspect of our lives was better—wasn't it? We gave more love to others, everything seemed easier, life was smoother, things bothered us less, and we were more relaxed, peaceful and more fulfilled. All because we saw the best in ourselves and loved ourselves!

It seems to me that when we are in love with another (but really ourselves), we are filled with joy, light and love—all qualities of God.

The layers of self-doubt are removed as that other person assures us we are special—and we believe we are special. We are totally connected to love (God) and this person, and feel safe and satisfied.

Consequently, our fears dissipate. We are full of hopeful expectations that we really believe (i.e., we have faith). We are not greedy because we feel fulfilled. We are generous—we feel we have an enormous capacity to give, and we give more freely.

This is the state of self-love. We need to hold this love for ourselves, because if we rely on another person for it, we are then dependent on another's feelings rather than thriving in the flow of God's unconditional love.

The person who loves us gives us a gift—a chance to experience what it is like to know and love our true selves. They are mirrors reflecting to us who we really are and what we can be! They teach us we are worthy of loving, despite the warts and all that bubbles up after we are out of the romantic phase of love.

There is a difference between "falling in love" and "stepping into" love. Falling implies a level of unconsciousness! We are not looking, and oops!—there we are. We have fallen in(to) love! And it feels great—we are in a giant vat of love! We are surrounded, supported and nourished by it and connected to everything.

And then someone plucks us out of the vat while we are unconscious of the fact that we have even been in a vat! We suddenly feel abandoned, desolate, alone and empty.

When someone plucks us out of the vat (i.e., they start to see our warts), self-doubt, a major enemy of self-love, creeps in. We are filled with fears—that we are not lovable, that there is something wrong with us (and they often tell us that too!), that we have baggage (who doesn't?)—self-judgments that make us miserable and convince us that we really are unworthy of love. Self-love and self-doubt both live in the heart. Your heart has to choose which one to follow!

Because we don't know how we ended up in, or out of, the vat of love, we can't consciously find our way back, and are bereft. God is that vat of love, and if we can learn to "step" into Him and His love, we can live in a state of reverence and love and sustain it.

Can you really feel what an astonishing being of light you are? (Okay, there are warts on the lights, but there are warts on *all* humans or we would not be human!)

Do you feel worthy of being loved—especially by yourself? Or will you allow your judgments, thoughts and fears convince you that you are unworthy, no good, ugly and flawed in so many ways that no one would want you?

Remember, fear is False Evidence Appearing Real! (I don't know who originally said that!)

Question the negative things you say to yourself or the fears you have. If there is some truth to them, then do something about changing! If there is no truth when you filter those ideas through your heart, block those thoughts out.

If everybody loved their true heart selves, there would be very few prisons, gangs, violence or cruelty in the world, because we all would treat ourselves—and everyone else—with love and reverence.

Say *Namaste* to yourself every morning in the mirror! Look into the mirror, look deeply into your eyes, and *see through* to your heart and say *Namaste* to your spirit. Listen for the gentle reply from the Divine.

P.S. If you are single, this all still applies to you! Even if you have never had an intimate relationship with anyone, you have had wonderful friendships where people have seen you as you really are, and you can use that as a starting place if you need to. Self-love starts with you—you don't need anyone else. Often people who are single and independent are very discerning and good at loving themselves anyway.

LOVE AND LIKE

I have learned that you can love someone and not like him or her very much!

When I am at my spiritual best and in my heart, I can do this very well. I am practicing sending love to people I don't particularly like—or whose actions, motives or intentions I don't like. (The latter is a more accurate statement.)

A lot of times you meet someone and instantly gel with them, and other times the opposite happens. Sometimes we sense a person's spirit (we *can* do it) and it doesn't gel with us. It may be wise to avoid them if possible. We are built to detect negative chemistry, electricity and magnetism. When we say, "I don't like so and so," we may be feeling mismatched chemistry or we may really be saying we don't like their morals or values, which are reflected in the way they behave or don't behave— for example, in how they treat others.

There is probably a bit of judgment thrown in there as well! (Just a bit!) Or even anger—this person has annoyed us so much and behaved so horribly *in our minds* that we just don't want to be anywhere near them.

When we say, "I don't like the way you are treating me right now," that is different from "I don't like YOU."

The solution is always the same—go to your heart and find love for them, or just put them in your heart and surround them with love. You don't have to like them or like what they do or be around them. Nor do you have to put up with what they are doing if it is abusive, violent or harmful. Remove yourself from the offending person, "place" them into your heart, *sincerely* surround them with love, and move on. Or away!

If you have to be around that person, do the "putting them into your heart and surrounding them with God's light and love" exercise; you will be amazed at how *they* seem different! This works *only* if you do this sincerely and gently with love and have no attachment to any outcome. All you are doing is holding them in your heart and allowing the alchemical magic of love to work on *you and them.*

This is a magical exercise! As a result of doing it, either we change, or they change, or everything changes because love is present. We are very gracious to everyone, including ourselves, when we have stepped into and live in the vat of love!

DAILY SCHEDULE
SUNDAY: **LOVE GOD**

"Thou shalt love the Lord thy God with all thy heart, and with all thy soul, and with all thy might. This is the first and great commandment."

—Matthew 22: 37,38

Love God first—and the rest will follow! It's your daily task for the rest of your life! Fill yourself with gratitude for God and all He does for us—that's one way to love Him!

One of the best ways to love God is to see Him in every person we meet and treat them the way He would. Can we put on "God glasses"? We would see the world through the eyes of God. Wouldn't that be awesome. If we could *really see* people as God sees them, I guess we would all be enlightened.

Before you think anything about anyone (or judge them), imagine you are looking at that person through God's eyes. We would see through to their astonishing light and beauty—past all the superficial attributes most of us normally look at—and we would respond with love and encouragement.

Encouragement may come in unexpected forms. Encouragement is not always positive or nurturing—it can be confronting and challenging and maybe even disciplining! Parents who never discipline their children or give them boundaries may not be doing the best thing.

Another way to love God is to spend time with Him. Not just on Sundays either! Each day, set aside some time to be quiet with Him. Better still, live the whole day aware of Him and connected to Him. Seek his counsel before you do anything major. Or minor! Ask him to be beside you all day, and ask Him for guidance with *all that you do.*

Ask what you can do to help God! We pray and ask God to help us, change things, do something or guide us. Or we pray when we are desperate and need a miracle, and when that miracle arrives, we go back to life as usual. That's not very reverent or loving, is it? Our memories are short! Ask Him to use you to help Him and to be a blessing others every day!

Being joyfully expectant of His answers and having patience and faith in God demonstrates our love in a different way. Keep on asking and listening. Love through listening to Him, then do what you feel He is guiding you to do.

Loving yourself is a way to love God—after all, we are part of Him and He us, and if we treat ourselves badly, we are treating God badly.

How does a parent feel if their child hates himself, is on drugs, or is harming himself in other ways? Horrible! If that child could love him- or herself, the parent would feel much better. I imagine that is what God would be like with us since He is our parent! It causes Him pain if we do not love ourselves and we treat ourselves badly. Like parents, He sees the gifts, grace and blessings we have been given. How sad when we are unaware of them.

There is a story (sorry, I don't know its source) about a man who was drowning in the ocean. He asked God to help him. Soon after, a ship came sailing by and the sailors called out, "We can save you." The drowning man responded, "No thanks—God has said He is going to save me. I'll wait." Then a submarine surfaced near him and sent out a rescue party. The man replied in the same way. Finally, as he was growing very tired, a helicopter flew over and lowered a man to pluck him out of the ocean, only to receive the same "No thanks" from the nearly drowned man.

Finally, the man did drown, and when he reached heaven, he said angrily to God, "Where were you? I was faithful and waited." God replied, "I sent you a ship, a submarine and a helicopter. What more could I do?"

God helps, but we also have to do our work, our part! We have to look for the angels He sends in all disguises, to wait patiently with joyful expectations for their arrival to actively listen for inspiration about what we need to do. Life isn't just handed to us on a platter—we have to do our part.

There are the times when we are just blessed with grace, but I suspect we receive more grace when we have tried hard to do what we believe God wants us to do.

Say your prayers with feeling and from your heart. Take a deep breath before you start speaking with God, and center yourself in your heart. Kneeling helps, as well! Repeating prayers that you know by heart and doing them without thought is better than nothing, but I suspect a heartfelt prayer that is like a gentle and humble conversation with God would be His preference! Be loving in your speech to Him and reverent in all that you say—to Him and others.

Trusting God demonstrates your love for Him. No matter what we feel is going on, and how bad things are, or what a mess we have gotten ourselves into, trust that you, with God's help or guidance, can somehow make good out of your mess or situation. Have faith in His goodness, kindness, grace and love.

Show God how you love Him today by trying to really feel that love in your heart. Be connected and open to Him so He can inspire you or comfort you. Allow Him to be close. If you are angry with Him, try to see the bigger picture. Be humble, be reverent and thank Him for all He has done for you.

Be grateful—very, very grateful. We can never comprehend how much we have been given. Be honest, open and completely in your heart when you are with God. Pray from your heart.

Send Him zoots!

MONDAY: BE A LOVE RAY-DIATOR! THINK ONLY LOVING THOUGHTS

"Today, greet every person inwardly as if they were wearing a sign on their forehead that says, 'God lives here.'"

—Mary Forte

Be conscious of this idea of God living in every other person and thing, and try to *feel* it before you speak to others. Be prepared to be stunned! You may just find that the whole world is happy today for no apparent reason. And *you* feel much more joyful. Doesn't that sound great?

Imagine that you have a stream of golden, white love light coming from the divine sun into the top of your head. It travels down to your heart, swirls around in the most magnificent patterns, fills up your heart, and then radiates out to surround you and others.

Try this in meetings, at dinner, at lunch, from your desk and as you drive. Practice it everywhere. (If you are driving, keep your eyes open!) It only takes a few seconds to do if your intentions are pure. And it is easy once you have practiced it. This makes you a "love *ray*-diator!"

This is another sign you could create for your house—"Be a love ray-diator!" Instead of giving children ray guns of the laser variety, we could give them love-ray guns! What if there were a toy shaped like a heart, and when you pressed it, it would radiate light!

Listen to what you say to yourself all day today. If your words are not loving, immediately replace them with loving or at least neutral words. Let nothing unloving come out of your mouth today, nor any *nonverbal* unloving messages! No rolling of the eyeballs or sighing, no snickering, sneering, slumping, shaking your head or closing your eyes in "quiet despair"! No thinking, "Here we go again" or "I knew this would happen!"

For your family, try especially hard today. Do nothing but love them and "ray" God's light over them! Keep them all in your heart—it's big enough! Shower them and surround them with light and love all day, and speak only lovingly to them. Encourage them and nurture them with your words and thoughts.

Focus on the good points of the people around you. Continually remind yourself of the positive, not the negative. Why do we focus long and hard on all the bad points and forget all the good points, when the loving thing is to do the opposite?

Today, there will be no sarcasm or preconceived expectations of difficulty or disappointment based on the past. Let go of that old stuff. It's a big day!

If you can do just a few of these things, it will be a great day!

See the sign on everyone's forehead—GOD LIVES HERE. Think only loving thoughts. See the I AM in everyone. Ban all judgment. Listen very carefully to what you say to yourself. Read nothing but up-

lifting, positive material. Watch only positive, uplifting television programs (this probably means turning the set off most of the time!). And
above all, bathe your family in your love.

TUESDAY: LOVING ACTIONS

"Love many things, for therein lies the true strength, and whoso-
ever loves much performs much and can accomplish much, and
what is done in love is done well."

—Vincent Van Gogh

Today is the day to be conscious of what you can *do* for others and how
you can serve them.

I often ask audiences, "Where do we learn to give love?" You should
see the blank looks in response!

We learn to give love from our parents. And our parents may have
struggled to show it in a way we could feel. When we meet the loves of
our lives, we don't ever discuss this—we just assume we know how to
show someone love, and we do, the way our family showed us. But the
person we're trying to love came from a completely different family and
they showed love in different ways.

Early in a relationship, this difference doesn't matter—but later on,
it can. We both think we are being loving to the other, but it's not the
loving they know. To prevent this scenario, ask this wonderful question,
"What do I do that makes you feel that I love you?" You too will be
greeted with a blank stare! But repeat the question and wait for the
answer. You may be surprised.

Once you ask this question and receive your answer, you are obliged
to do what they ask! If you are not prepared to do that, then don't ask
the question. Ask your children as well—it is a fabulous way to teach
them love and for you to learn what makes them feel loved. You may be
surprised at the answers!

Do what they tell you with joy and reverence. If you do it begrudg-
ingly or grit your teeth and tell yourself, "I can't *believe* I am doing

this!"—it is NOT love. Remember, loving is all about giving—you are *freely* giving something that you know makes them feel loved.

Anybody you help is receiving your love. Find people to help today. Ask them if they would *like* your help first! That is one of my "little" learning points—to wait for people to ask me for help before I do it! I struggle a lot with that, so I *know it is a major lesson.*

I really do believe there are times when we can give gifts in the form of help without being asked—like doing something that really needs to be done for our parents, friends or partner if they have not had time to do it. We could take out the garbage for an elderly neighbor, mow their lawn or shovel their snow. We could do the same for our parents.

I mentioned earlier that, in retrospect, this was a tough lesson I learned with Mama. How I wish now that I had sat with her and loved her instead of running around "helping" her by doing the shopping, cleaning, cooking and other stuff. Maybe we help more sometimes by just sitting with someone and surrounding them with love and light, and talking and laughing with them. I suspect we do. I wish I had.

Learn from me and go straight out and call your elderly parent or parents, talk with them and tell them what is going on in your life. Or just sit, be with them and love them. Invite them to talk about their favorite things. Listen to the same old stories with love and *interest* (this is *really* loving!). Be present with them. Cry with them. Laugh with them. Share your life with them. Talk to them and let them feel they are a part of your life—an important part!

Be present when you are there—you are not giving them *heart time* if your mind is somewhere else. Your heart and mind need to be with them completely for you to really be actively loving them.

Affection and hugging is a powerful way to show love! *Any* kind of loving gesture or touch—even a loving look—can change someone's day. Sending zoots is another great way to give love!

Volunteering is another way of acting out love; so are mentoring and teaching. Anything where we *serve* another is love in action. A person is never really happy unless he or she is serving.

Call a friend who is having a tough time. Or call someone you have not spoken to for a while and say, "Hello, I am thinking of you." Leave a little love note under the pillow for your children or partner. Smile at strangers. Be thoughtful—think about what others would like or what would make them happy. Write a letter telling someone how special they are to you and mail it to them. Spread little heart confetti around someone's desk! There are hundreds of little loving actions you can do every day.

Be creative. DO something loving today!

WEDNESDAY: LOVE YOUR LIFE

> "I am not sure exactly what heaven will be like, but I do know that when we die and it comes time for God to judge us, He will NOT ask, 'How many good things have you done in your life?' Rather He will ask, 'How much LOVE did you put into what you did?'"
>
> —Mother Teresa

Do you love your life? Really love it? When someone asks, "How are you?" can you answer with an enthusiastic, "I *LOVE* my life!"

If not—today is the day to start.

So many people grumble and moan about what they have to do, how horrible their job is and how hard life is. Hmmmm, I wonder, what's the alternative? Imagine how much you would love this life of yours if you were told you only had three months to live!

If you are the sort of person who would not change a thing in your life with this news, be thankful. Most people would make some changes, and often, they would be significant changes. Most certainly they would start to savor all the moments—no matter how challenging! Or they would let go of grudges, issues of control or irritations, realizing that's the "small stuff," and they would stop wasting precious time being angry or annoyed. They would concentrate more on loving and spending time with people they love and on the really important *things* in life—which of course are not "things"!

Your life has made you what you are. When people want to change the past, I wonder if it means they don't like themselves. You are the person you are *because* you went through those things. Blaming the past is like driving with a huge rearview mirror in front of you: you can see only what has passed and not what lies ahead.

We *always* have a choice in our lives—and before you cry, "No, I didn't!" consider this very, very carefully! Somewhere there will be one, or many, points where you made a decision to move in the direction of this life you are currently living. If *you* got you here, then *you* can get you out of here!

If you hate your job and can't find purpose and meaning in what you are doing, then leave! If you can't leave, then make it your mission to be an outstanding employee, no matter what your job entails. Just doing that will give you a sense of pride and shift your focus so your job becomes more satisfying. Find all the good parts of the job and focus on the blessings the job gives you—such as financial security or medical insurance or interaction with great people.

Our jobs fill the majority of our lifetime, so make sure you choose to enjoy yours and experience a sense of fulfillment from it. If you grumble and hate every minute of what you do each day, not only do you become an energy sucker and alienate everyone, but you ruin your chances of enjoyment, promotion or recognition. You also give nothing or contribute little, and deep down, you feel bad about yourself. Aim to be the best you can be at whatever it is that you are doing.

What about loving your life even if it needs changing? Find something to love about it and focus on that part until the changes are in place. Love your current life, as it is sure to be giving you great lessons. Be grateful for it. Search through it for the divine gifts it bears.

If you have decided you want a new life or want to modify your current one, be patient. It may be that you have to learn some lessons while in this job or relationship before you can move on. What you think you *want* may not always be what you actually *need*, and God knows the right time for everything. (Maybe He's waiting for you to make the most of what you have before He gives you something else!)

In other words, love what you have. It may need changing, but focus on the good things about your life as you arrange for the changes to occur. Stop looking in the rearview mirror. Do your *work*. Love your life.

THURSDAY: GIVE EVERYONE TA-DA'S!

"The little unremembered acts of kindness and love are the best parts of a person's life."

—William Wordsworth

This is another day to make others feel great! Don't you love your life? Your mission is to see all the silent TA-DA's today.

Everybody wants acceptance, recognition and acknowledgment. They are primary motivating forces in life, both at work and at home. People want to be, and feel, accepted. Why do people join gangs or have affairs? Why do some children blossom and excel at school and in life, when just *one* teacher takes an interest in them? If just *one* person at work cares about or takes an interest in us and what we are doing, why do we find ourselves performing better and trying harder?

All these things happen because of needing recognition and acknowledgment of *who* we are as much as *what* we have done. It is one of the most powerful forms of motivation and is one of the ways we "wrap" others in love.

After one of my presentations, a man named Roger from Wisconsin shared with me a story about visiting his sister, who had a four-year-old son. This little boy asked Uncle Roger to come and watch him at his gymnastics competition. The little boy was walking on a balance beam, which was about an inch off the ground, as he was only four! He jumped off the end in triumph and threw his hands up in the air and shouted "TA-DA!"

Isn't that wonderful? Of course all the adults clapped and cheered. All toddlers love doing anything that generates attention, so they are all masters of doing TA-DA's!

Writing one of my monthly email newsletters on this topic, I realized that we all love doing TA-DA's until about age eight, when it becomes "uncool" to do them out loud! But I believe we all keep doing silent TA-DA's on the inside. We are closet TA-DAists! Every time we do something of which we are proud or pleased, *inside* we are jumping up and shouting "TA-DA!"

The trouble is, most people don't see these silent TA-DA's and we feel de-motivated or disappointed. We *must* look for people's silent TA-DA's! It is the single most motivating thing we can do—to notice them, look for them, listen for them and say, "I think that deserves a TA-DA!" Watch their faces glow and spirits shine when you do notice, because you just gave some love and inspired them to go out and be even better.

This is a brilliant management, leadership or parenting tip! See and acknowledge others' TA-DA's. Give yourself TA-DA's!

Today, recognize TA-DA's in at least three people. Be on the lookout for those moments when they are telling you something that could deserve a TA-DA!—it may be very small, so listen carefully. Say, as often as you can, "I think that deserves a TA-DA!" and enjoy the response. Look for opportunities to acknowledge someone. Make a generous comment about someone's children—there are always opportunities for TA-DA's!

Create a TA-DA culture at your workplace. Have TA-DA awards. Let people nominate the person of the month who deserves a TA-DA! Talk about TA-DA's at staff meetings. Create opportunities for people to deserve TA-DA's!

Give people sincere compliments. Tell them they are looking great (and mean it!) or that they have done a wonderful job, or tell them something you sincerely appreciate about them or what they do for you, others or their work. Comment on a quality you admire in them—there are a thousand ways of making someone feel special.

Give yourself a TA-DA for doing all this!

FRIDAY: LOVE YOURSELF

"Your task is not to seek for love but merely to seek and find all the barriers within yourself that you have built against it."

—Rumi

Wake up and walk straight to the mirror today and say *Namaste* to yourself! Today is the day you find your incredible I AM spirit!

Reread the section on loving yourself above, and go through today seeing yourself from your heart's perspective and not your judgment's! No negative or destructive self-talk today! Not one word—only goodness, kindness, compassion and tenderness with yourself.

Give yourself a break—even if no one else does! Allow yourself TA-DA's!—acknowledge them yourself and compliment *yourself* on a job well done if you have to. Allow yourself to make mistakes without berating yourself. Understand you're doing your best and if you could do it better, you would. In other words, give yourself grace.

Be the person that is in your true heart. Follow your heart's "knowings"—they are not emotions or feelings but knowings. Your criticizer gives you all the facts, reasons, judgments and nasty stuff! Your true heart only gives you wisdom and truth. Ask your heart today what you need to do to find self-love, what barriers you need to remove. Listen carefully and then do it.

Love your body even if it is not in perfect shape. (After all, whose is?) Treat it well today. Take time to truly nourish it with lovingly prepared food instead of shoving any old processed fast food in, as quickly and unconsciously as you can.

Today, find ways to give yourself joy. Do all the things a loving parent would do for you! You may not have had a loving parent, but you will have seen how other loving parents behave, so treat yourself like that today. Be patient, kind, caring, nurturing, understanding and compassionate and hug yourself!

See if you can make your own eyes sparkle with inspiration, motivation or enthusiasm today! What or who inspires you? Spend time with them or read about them today. What motivates you? Spend some time doing that today. Pursue your passion in some way and notice how you feel. If you don't have a passion, find one! Begin the search now.

Be enthusiastic today, even if you are generally not an enthusiastic person. It's fun and a way to express an exuberant side of your personality! Even if you surprise people and they say, "What have you done with the old (insert your name here)?" laugh and say, "This is who is inside the old me!"

Love yourself enough to be real and authentic in front of others—be who you really are, and if they don't like it, too bad for them!

When we find the seed of I AM inside us and allow that to shine forth, it is the real us and we are incredibly loving and lovable. Go ahead—love yourself, be the real you, and watch your world change!

SATURDAY: HOLD PEOPLE IN YOUR HEART

"Today, see if you can stretch your heart and expand your love so that it touches not only those to whom you can give it easily but also to those who need it so much."[2]

—Daphne Rose Kingma

I have mentioned that the heart rules all the other organs and functions of the body. Most people think that the brain is the most important organ for life, but they are wrong! Once the heart stops, life stops. People can be brain dead and still alive. In fact, many people walk around like that every day! Make sure you are not one of them. Be conscious of the power and beauty of your heart today.

The alchemical capacities of the heart are to love, heal, forgive and change everything. To tap into this alchemy, we have to hold people in our hearts.

Think of someone with whom you would like to have a better relationship, or someone who is causing you a lot of grief or pain in your life. Create an image of them or sense their qualities and "place" them inside your heart.

I have mentioned the technique before but I want to repeat it here so you don't have to look back: Sit quietly and imagine there is a tunnel going from the top of your head to the inside of your heart—like a water chute. Place this person into the top of the chute and gently slide them down to the interior of your heart—which is very spacious! Allow them to be there for a moment or so. (If it feels really good, keep them there as long as you like.) While you hold that person in your heart, all the love and light that lives in the heart caresses them and gives them whatever they need. You have no intention other than to be a blessing and keep them in your heart, so it can work its magic.

Notice how you feel while you are doing this. There is usually a sense of peace that settles on you as your heart works on you, as well! If you want to, after you have done this, you can imagine your heart kind of turning inside out and *ray*-ing out like those religious paintings of Christ and Mary. As you gently ray these light forces out, the person floats out in front of you on those rays and you can "see" them in front of you surrounded by this beautiful light. The first time I did this at a Sacred Service class, the light was a gorgeous pink and then after that, it was golden, white or both!

This might sound very New Age and cosmic, but I promise it is not. I learned how to do this heart work with Robert and Cheryl Sardello, and I have actually seen, felt, heard and experienced profound changes in both myself and others. I just need to remind myself to do it more often—like all humans, I am so busy trying to do things to improve circumstances, I forget *the most powerful thing to do* is hold others in my heart!

If I have a business meeting, I do this before the meeting and I do it before I speak, always. You can hold a lot of people in your heart!

You are making a commitment today that you will remember to put people in your heart *before you do anything else!*

It should be awesome!

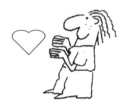

CHAPTER 11

A WEEK OF **CHEERFUL ENTHUSIASM**

"A cheerful spirit is one of the most valuable gifts ever bestowed upon humanity by a kind Creator. It will hold in check the demons of despair, and stifle the power of discouragement and hopelessness."

— James H. Aughey

YOUR **SEVEN MINUTES**

Are you a cheerful person?

Are you an enthusiastic person?

Are you passionate about something that you whole-*heart*-edly believe in?

Are you optimistic?

Do you feel your life has purpose and meaning?

If not, why not? You are not allowed to blame anybody or any thing! *You* are taking responsibility for your life as it is right now—so what is it *in you* that has blocked any of the above? Beliefs? Thoughts? Fears? Expectations? Living in the past? Judgments? Other things?

Make a few notes about what might be blocking you and what you can do about it.

AMANDA'S TAKE ON CHEERFUL ENTHUSIASM

"If you are not getting as much from life as you want to, then examine the state of your enthusiasm."

—Norman Vincent Peale

IT'S ALWAYS SUNNY ABOVE THE CLOUDS

"It's Always Sunny Above the Clouds" is the name of an article I wrote after a plane ride. We took off from a dark and gloomy airport, burst through the cloud barrier (notice the words!) and found magnificent, cloudless blue skies with sunshine that streamed into the windows of the plane. It dawned on me that every time I have left a cloudy, stormy place on the ground, it's always been sunny above the clouds!

Think of the number of times we speak of people who have a "sunny disposition." Everyone knows that means they are cheerful and joyful. The sun is very important in cheerfulness—more than we know or remember. There is even a medical condition called SAD—seasonal affective disorder—that influences people's moods during months of limited sunlight. We are also learning how important the sun is for vitamin D and other physiological needs.

The Inca and other ancient cultures understood the value of the sun to the point where they actually worshipped it and believed it was responsible for their abundance. They had the ability to perceive the spirit of the sun as approachable and incredibly powerful, and they asked it to bring goodness, health and crops. They were thankful for its warmth and spirit of protection, and believed that their king was a descendent of the sun who would look after them in the same ways.

The Bible also tells us to be like the sun, shining in people's lives.

Spend time in the sun each sunny day and thank it for beaming all that warmth, light and life into your body and spirit. Without the sun, there would be no life on earth. Living our first winter in Vermont sure taught me the value of the warmth in sunlight—it's amazing!

A few days of rain, mist, cold, snow and clouds leave most people feeling gloomy—just like the weather. As soon as the sun and its warmth and light emerge again, our spirits soar.

Imagine what life would be like if we all aimed to have a sunny disposition, to be cheerful no matter what clouds were about, remembering that clouds also give life-giving rain and shade, and to be filled with gratitude, seeking the gifts of the clouds and the sun—both inner and outer!

The clouds can represent the trials and tribulations—learning opportunities—in life. Once we move past them, break or burst through them—we find the sun again. Or we can find a haven in the little breaks between the clouds—the little patches of sunlight. Isn't that a great way to look at our life struggles—as a cloud cover that eventually passes?

The Bridge Over the River is a great book written by the sister of a young soldier named Sigwart who was killed in World War 1. The sister believed she was able to communicate with her brother after his death. (This book has been translated by Joseph Wetzl.)

Sigwart gives many great words of advice from the heavenly realms that have struck chords with me. For example, he says we should "bear all discomforts cheerfully" and that our spirit welcomes upsets because it knows they are for its benefit. By working through our clouds or discomforts—learning our lessons, strengthening our will and soul—we can grow and develop into more spiritual human beings. Our challenge is to see the clouds as the gifts they are!

WHAT IS REALLY CAUSING YOUR GLOOM?

When "clouds" are present in our life, we can feel gloomy, sad, burdened, heavy and hopeless. It can seem like a fog at times; things are dark or dreary and murky no matter where we look, but our ability to see clearly or understand the whole is limited.

Gloom comes mostly from unclear thinking, when we give in to negative emotions or self talk, or our perceptions are skewed, inaccurate or just plain wrong! (Of course the gloom I am talking about here is not clinical depression or any other physiological or medical condition.)

Gloom is the opposite of feeling enthusiastic, sunny, alive and joyful. This whole book is dedicated to eliminating gloom and giving us more control over our moods. As you work your way through the exercises, you can decide which ones help you soar through the clouds to God's sunshine above.

STORMS

Storms come in all sorts of shapes and sizes. They can be huge, swirling, scary, tumultuous thunderstorms that suddenly appear out of nowhere, or they can just be heavy, solid, consistent rain or snow that sets in for days. There may even be hail and tornadoes or "willy willys" as we call them in Australia!

But no matter what type of storm we face, the sun returns. We may be changed or may have to recover from damage sustained during the storm, but if we are resilient, cheerful and optimistic, if we choose to think with a joyful heart that things will improve, we move forward more quickly.

JENI

One particular young woman I know suffered through a monster storm. Jeni was a perfectly healthy 32-year-old in a new marriage, but she was not feeling well and thought she was pregnant. A local physician diagnosed her with the flu. Several days later, she collapsed and was rushed to the intensive care unit with septicemia—her whole body was poisoned.

For seven weeks, she was in intensive care, with a wonderful supportive family around her praying. It did not look good, and people thought only a miracle would help her.

And a miracle did happen—she lived, but the damage that had ravaged her body meant she had to have both legs amputated just below the knee and both hands amputated. She, her family and her doctors were all very excited and enthusiastic because *they were able to save her wrists*. Makes you think differently, doesn't it?

Continuing on her journey to come off the respirator and start using a badly traumatized body that had not moved for seven weeks, she had to work extremely hard. Her physical therapist said she had never seen anyone so enthusiastic or cheerful about her exercises—all of which involved a lot of pain.

People who suffer major trauma like this are in danger of adopting a "victim" mentality. They cannot move past their injuries or escape thinking, "Poor me, why me, this is unfair, life is not worth living," even after a significant time of healing. They can become trapped in self-centeredness, depression, anger and fear.

But that's not Jeni! She defied death and now she is using her sunny, cheerful spirit as a beacon for others—she is *giving* to others instead of wallowing in depression. The first time she left the hospital was to a McDonald's with her dad. People stared at her, but her only concern was how the experience was affecting her dad!

When she went to visit the surgeon who had to do the amputations, her main objective was to reassure him that she was okay: she knew how emotionally difficult it had been for him to operate on her. She is a truly incredible, compassionate spirit—*she* was the one without hands and feet, and all she did was care for others and reassure them that everything was great.

The thought of life without feet and hands would be a big challenge for me, but not Jeni. She is brave, strong and, most importantly, optimistic. She has a wonderful, supportive, loving husband and family who adore her. Everyone who knows her and meets her is in awe of her enthusiastic spirit and her will to move on and start her new life, which, I might add, includes children, writing and speaking, and running her own foundation for children with disabilities.

Jeni epitomizes another Sigwart quotation: "Tread smilingly on the most difficult paths. In your will lies the strength of fulfillment. Never let thoughts of doubt arise in you. These are great obstacles."[1]

Neither doubt, nor fear, nor any other obstacle will stop Jeni!

Here is another example of the power of her spirit. I had sent an email asking about her health to Jeni's best friend (and one of mine), Somer. Her reply highlights Jen'is inspirational spirit:

"She is doing well and is unbelievably content. She had physical therapy last night while I was there and they worked on making a tool so she could turn pages in a magazine. I asked if that made her feel sad or dependent. She enthusiastically replied that it was quite the opposite; it made her feel liberated and independent. That was a huge lesson for me—almost like the glass-half-full thing—but putting myself in her shoes, it truly showed me what kind of person I was and how I look at things."

Somer is an inspiration as well. She has battled her own obstacle-filled journey with grace and cheerfulness. Life does not come without obstacles—they are an important part of the journey. *The spirit* in which we deal with these obstacles makes all the difference in our lives.

Learning about Jeni's amazing spirit has helped me a great deal to put whatever I *thought* were challenges into perspective. Every day when you are feeling grumpy or gloomy, recall her story and use her spirit as a beacon for yours. Her spirit is calling you to the sunshine and asking you to cheerfully look at something currently worrying you. Reframing a challenge helps us to see it as a necessary growth opportunity and a blessing—yes, a *blessing*!

Find the gifts in the obstacles you face. How you face them determines whether you find the gift or not. Jeni not only found her gifts but is showering others with them.

From Sigwart: *"The greatness of a human being depends on how much he carries the sun in himself."*[2]

Jeni is truly great.

THE ORIGIN OF ENTHUSIASM

"Years may wrinkle the skin, but to give up enthusiasm wrinkles the soul."

—Samuel Ullman

The Greek root of the word "enthusiasm" is *en-theos*—*en* meaning "in" or "see," and *theos* meaning "God." Enthusiasm means "having the God within" or "seeing the God within." It shines from people who are filled with light, life and God's love.

People with enthusiasm, who are motivated, passionate, inspired or in love, always have wonderful, bright, vital, sparkling eyes! It makes them very attractive to everyone. Perhaps it's the magic of a spirit coming alive that makes our eyes sparkle?

That's your mission, should you choose to accept it! Put a sparkle into the eyes of every single person you meet! Share your light with others. Spread your enthusiasm.

If you don't believe you have light within you, your mission is to search for it or ask for help finding it. It *is* there! The key is to find God and the divine worlds inside and around you and let that unlock you so the light will shine into and through you! Spend time with people like Jeni, serve others, and you will find that light. Focus on goodness, kindness, compassion and gratitude, and then God's light will brighten inside you.

When we are connected with God, we are filled with enthusiasm, and feel peaceful, joyful, excited *and exciting* all at the same time.

A PASSION FOR BEING ENTHUSIASTIC

"The real secret of success is enthusiasm."

—Walter Chrysler

How alive do you feel right now? What sorts of things make you feel alive? What gives your life meaning? What purpose do you have for this lifetime or at this time in your life? What makes you feel passionate?

These are all critical questions for building enthusiasm and joy.

Having a passion for something makes it easier to be enthusiastic, but I think we are meant to be enthusiastic about *everything*, not just what we have a passion for. Why not be passionate about being enthusiastic or connecting with God and being full of light and life? Or being passionate and enthusiastic about being alive?

No matter what your life is like, there is always the opportunity to change. Neuroscience teaches us that we *can* re-hardwire our brains— and we know God can change our hearts. There is always a chance to grow and develop or be free of old beliefs, to learn, to be forgiven, to forgive, to stop old patterns, to lighten up, to rethink and to reframe. There is still time *while you are alive to learn your lessons!*

Develop your will forces and courage, and embrace whatever it is you have to do to enjoy your life. Clear your thinking, find your true heart, live from your heart, see the bigger spiritual picture—there are so many exciting possibilities! I feel enthusiastic just typing this!

I will never forget a woman I met years ago and loved being around. She was the most vibrant and enthusiastic person. She told me that when she was growing up, her mother would put enthusiasm into everything. She would say in a really excited voice, "Let's do the washing up!" and this little girl would say in an equally enthusiastic voice, "OKAY!" And then they would both embark with gusto on washing up. My friend now does this with her children and it's a great lesson. Children model what they see, hear and feel. What are you teaching your children?

My wonderful mother must have done that for me, as I never tackle anything halfheartedly! I don't drag myself out to do stuff I have to do. I may not always be as cheerful as I could be, but I am enthusiastic to have it all done, so I am more focused and efficient and do more.

I notice that when I am with my godchildren, my spirit is fired with enthusiasm and I love it! Isabella will say to me, "Let's play!" and I say, like the seven-year-old she is, "Great! What will we play?" And soon we are just rolling in excitement, enthusiasm and laughter! I cannot begin to describe the blessings and joy that little girl gives me.

Small children cry, laugh, play, sing and dance with the greatest enthusiasm—they are naturally alive. Then they grow older and enthusiasm becomes uncool. Most teenagers have replaced enthusiasm with disdain, and most adults are too drained to be enthusiastic. They do not choose to give themselves time to renew or restore their connection with God and their life forces.

Remember, real enthusiasm is felt when we *feel* the Divine inside us—when we feel it in each of our cells and it shines out of us. If we remind ourselves to do *everything* we do with God's love in our hearts, and feel God with us, then our enthusiasm will make us sparkle. *Feel* God first. Then *do*!

MEANING AND PURPOSE IN LIFE, OR WORK VS. A JOB

Things that give our lives meaning and purpose will ignite the sparks of joyful enthusiasm inside us.

We rarely have a deep sense of fulfillment and satisfaction from *just* making money or buying material possessions. That may give us some short-term happiness but nothing deep or sustaining. For deep, abiding, fulfilling satisfaction, we need to be working with something—either at work or on our own time—that inspires us and gives our life meaning and purpose. Find your purpose. Seek some meaning in what you do—create it if you need to.

Think about what inspired you as a child. What excited you? What did you love to learn about? What did you love to do?

There may be activities that make you feel wonderful, like swing dancing, painting, playing a musical instrument, reading, learning, playing tennis or hiking. These can make you feel great short-term, but they do not give you abiding fulfillment unless you can find a way to combine the activity you love with doing something for the world or others—some form of serving.

Perhaps you could become a teacher of swing or another form of dancing and share the joy of it with others while helping them become fit at the same time. Or you could teach any of the things that you love to do and help others share your enthusiasm.

You can even turn tedious tasks into playful activities to generate enthusiasm. Sing as you clean, or make what you are doing into a game and celebrate when you finish.

There is a big difference between "a job" and "work." Our work is what we are *meant* to be doing—the work of developing ourselves, serving and loving others, and making our own unique contribution to the universe. Can you combine your *work* with your job?

HOW I FELL INTO SPEAKING: MY PURPOSE

I am so blessed that God led me to a path where I do what I love. I feel I have a strong purpose and there is great meaning to what I do. Being a speaker combines my work and my job. I had little to do with it, mind you! It was through grace more than anything that I "fell" into speaking!

I was a physical therapist working in ergonomics and occupational health. I had coauthored a book, which prompted a meeting planner to invite me to a conference where inspirational speaker Ron Tacchi was the emcee.

At the end of my presentation, Ron said, "You should be a speaker!" and I answered, "What's a speaker?" He then mentored me into the business, which in itself was a huge blessing, as he is one of the best speakers I have ever heard.

I am humbled when I consider how God has orchestrated, and been my guide through, an amazing and wonderful career that has allowed me to travel to many countries. I am blessed to feel He makes a difference through me. I love my work—and I work diligently to do what I believe He wants me to do.

DO YOUR BEST AND ENTHUSIASM GROWS

Disliking your job is not healthy for you or those with whom you work. Challenge yourself to make the job fun or to do it better than it has ever been done. Use your intellect to find ways to make that possible—

few things make you more enthusiastic or are more motivating than challenging yourself. With this approach, your job may become your work, changing *you*! You will be noticed and your character and enthusiasm will make you attractive for promotions. More importantly, you will feel better about yourself.

If your meaning in life comes from other than your job, still do your job the very best you can. Be honest, operate with integrity and loyalty, do the right thing by everyone, including yourself and be cheerful, and you will be surprised at how enthusiasm appears and grows in your life.

WHAT INSPIRES YOU?

Consider for a few minutes the times when you have been really enthusiastic in life. What were the circumstances? Can you find factors in those circumstances that are common, that might give you clues as to the qualities of things that fire you up? In your conversations, what topics make you literally wake up? If you begin a conversation feeling tired and flat and finish feeling wide awake, excited and cheerful, then you have a big clue!

What are your values and what is important in life for you? It is my nature to be curious and I love to learn. In fact, learning is my number-one value and I find if I am not learning, some part of my spirit shrivels. I can do almost anything, anywhere, as long as I am learning.

Explore your values and see what information they give about what gives your life meaning and purpose and lights your fires of enthusiasm!

SERVING OTHERS

Really, everything we do, *everything*, should be about *serving others*. We are happiest when we are serving others. Whether you are working with customers, your bosses, colleagues, other companies, the community, the world or the shareholders, try to be of service. Serving others in less fortunate situations reminds us just how blessed we are and how joy is not dependent on material possessions.

If we can look at every aspect of our lives as a form of service to others, purpose, meaning and cheerful enthusiasm will flow freely. While we metaphorically "wash the feet of others," we feed our hearts and souls. It's a win-win.

MIRACLES

If the opportunities to consciously grow and develop don't excite you or make you feel cheerful, then consider the miraculous!

Austrian philosopher and playwright Rudolf Steiner, in a lecture called "The Work of the Angel in Our Astral Body," says, "We must get into the habit of being alert. . . . If we do not discover a miracle in our life on a particular day, we have merely lost sight of it." He suggests that every night we ask ourselves (and it would be a fun thing to do with someone else, as well), "What might have happened to me today?"

Then look for the "mini" miracles, which is what I call them. Major miracles happen every day to someone somewhere, but miracles are not usually of that magnitude every day in our lives. *However, mini miracles do happen every day.*

Imagine you are running out the door to make an appointment, but someone turns up at your house and delays you. This makes you annoyed, stressed and tense and ruins your day. Reflect on this event in the evening. Who knows if an angel orchestrated the delay so that you avoided the car crash you would have been involved in had you left on time? Thinking like this transforms your perceptions and life.

If a disappointing interview or decision at work had been successful, perhaps it would have put you in a job you hated and that made you miserable.

Missing a plane, which put you into a foul mood for the day, could have saved your life. We never know because we never see the whole.

In other words, before you sleep, look at what you deem "negative" aspects of your life, and knowing there is a wise guidance behind them, find the blessings within. Try to be conscious of this higher wisdom by doing this fun exercise! It makes the end of the day a much more cheerful and miraculous experience!

MOODS AND YOU

Which brings me back to moods.

Who is in charge of your mood? Of course, it's you! Only you can be responsible for how you react, and although your feelings can be hurt, you can manage your hurt emotions with cheerfulness or activity or by doing something to make yourself feel better.

I am the sort of person who warns others about how I feel. If I know it is "that" time of the month or I don't feel well or I am very tired and I know I am more likely to be grumpy or difficult, I warn people. I say, "This has nothing to do with you, but I am feeling sick right now or blah, blah, blah."

I have to remind myself that *my* mood is *my* choice and I have the resources to change it and be happier or more enthusiastic. I try to exercise my will and be cheerful. Sometimes I can, but if I am really tired, I find it difficult. So I take responsibility, warn others and try to do the things I need to do to return to a cheerful and enthusiastic state. Like sleep!

Are you willing to take charge of how you feel and your moods and smile your way through everything? Or at least treat other people well and not make them suffer because *you* are tired, miserable or angry?

One thing that can help a great deal is to say, "I am *experiencing* or *feeling* depressed/angry/frustrated right now"—not "*I am* depressed/angry/frustrated." This is a small change but it has a profound effect. If you say, "*I AM* depressed, etc." you are downloading that negative pattern into all of your cells. You are *owning* it, becoming it and maintaining it.

BAD-MOOD BUSTERS

♥ Connect to your heart. (The heart is never in a bad mood!)
♥ Exercise to release endorphins. (Check with a doctor if you don't usually do this, and just move as much as the doctor deems prudent.)
♥ Do some breathing exercises.

♥ Smile—even a fake smile releases endorphins!

♥ Watch a funny movie.

♥ Listen to what you are saying to yourself, and change anything negative to positive.

♥ Learn something new.

♥ Go and visit a hospice or somewhere where you can serve someone who is less fortunate than you.

♥ Think of Jeni and stop feeling sorry for yourself.

♥ Laugh even if you don't feel like it.

♥ Read uplifting books, listen to uplifting CDs or watch uplifting DVDs.

♥ Call a good friend and talk about good times.

♥ Look through or create a photo album of happy times.

♥ Walk in nature. Absorb the wonderful vibrations from the flowers, trees, grass, rocks and water and anything beautiful you find there!

♥ Make a gratitude list of all the blessings in your life and those things for which you are grateful.

♥ Look for the miracles in your day before you go to sleep.

There are a million ways to let off steam. Take responsibility and just do something to find more joy!

ARE YOU A SPIRIT IGNITER OR A SPIRIT PHOOFER?

I believe that everyone we meet has a pilot light inside them—just like a gas stovetop. By turning a switch on the stove we can ignite that flame or extinguish it. All of us have a choice with people—we can ignite their inner flame or light, or blow it out with a single breath. We can make another person's day or extinguish their spirit with a word, smile, look or gesture.

There are "spirit igniters" and "spirit phoofers." The phoofers blow out that pilot light the way we would blow out a candle. Most of us have had moments where we have phoofed out someone's spirit! Hopefully this book will show you how to be an igniter and never be a phoofer again!

Spirit igniters have eyes that sparkle with excitement, enthusiasm and joy, and that radiate over everyone they encounter, in turn lighting other spirits and making them sparkle!

Spirit phoofers can blow out your spirit with one nasty glance or cutting word! Haven't you met someone like that? Someone who looks at you or speaks to you in such a tone that your spirit immediately shrivels up?

Make it a goal to ignite someone's spirit each day. A person whose spirit has shriveled has eyes that are listless and lifeless. Their eyes don't sparkle, twinkle, dance or smile. Help these people just by being your sparkling, igniting self around them!

If it's your habit to behave as a spirit phoofer—catch yourself, laugh at yourself and change! You might even say, "I'm sorry, I didn't mean to do that."

CELEBRATE

Another way to keep enthusiasm alive is to celebrate! Celebrate not just major life events but also the little ones. Celebrate that you have your health, a car, and a roof over your head—or not! Celebrate the sunrise or the sunset. Celebrate the onset of spring or any other season. Celebrate that you lost a pound! Celebrate by yourself and with others!

Doing a little celebration dance or singing a song works just as well as large expensive events! I know this sounds silly, but we need to find small ways to celebrate that touch our hearts. Give someone a TA-DA! Tell them they deserve a TA-DA and watch their spirit sparkle! Give yourself a TA-DA and do it in front of the mirror! Smile at yourself and say, "Well done!" Celebrate just by feeling good and enjoying that feeling. Or celebrate by slowing down for a few minutes, just sitting and enjoying a view or a quiet moment.

Find small and meaningful ways to celebrate more frequently, so that life is a series of mini celebrations rather than a series of disappointments, struggles or difficulties. This helps us maintain a cheerful attitude in the face of everything that comes our way.

SMILE—WITH JOY

There is a Tibetan saying, "When you smile at life, half the smile is for your face; the other half is for someone else's."

Isn't that true? There are so many songs about smiling, particularly the song that says, "When you smile, the whole world smiles with you."

What happens to our face when a baby or toddler smiles at us? We smile back! Even if a grown-up smiles at us, our natural tendency is to smile back.

How sad it is that it often gives us a surprise or shock when we look up and someone is smiling at us. What has happened that we are so disconnected from everyone that we are uncomfortable if someone gives us a sincere and genuine smile from the heart? Many of us immediately wonder what that person is smiling at, or worse, why they are smiling at us. In fact, it may be just that someone had a happy thought and their face automatically showed it with a smile, and you were blessed enough to be one of the recipients.

There are a lot of different smiles out there. Some people mistake a smile for a grimace! Or they smile and their eyes don't smile, so it does not seem like a smile. Think of all the different types of smiles you have experienced—and given!

The best smile for me is the smile that radiates out of someone's cheerful heart—and especially a smile from a young child. Their eyes sparkle and their whole face is full of joy. Those smiles make your spirit sparkle so brightly that others will need sunglasses!

Smiles cost nothing and give a great deal more than we can quantify—both to ourselves and to others. We actually release endorphins (the body's natural happy drugs) with a large grin. We can release them any time we like by laughing or smiling sincerely.

Put a giant grin on your face, feel the smile in your heart and make your eyes smile as well, and you will be releasing endorphins!

Share your smiles today!

DAILY SCHEDULE

SUNDAY: LOOK FOR MIRACLES

"It's faith in something and enthusiasm for something that makes life worth living."

—Oliver Wendell Holmes

Today your mission is to see miracles wherever you look!

Of course the easiest place to see miracles is in nature. Consider the miracle of the bumblebee. Engineers tell us it cannot fly according to the laws of aerodynamics—but it does. Or consider the plants that burst (literally) into life after being buried by snow for six months. Consider the way the sun comes up every day and the oceans flow; the way small plants find a crack, take root and grow in the concrete jungles of our cities. All of nature is miraculous.

And so are people. The miracles of caring, creativity, kindness, compassion and resilience happen every minute somewhere. So does the miracle of healing, not to mention the miracles that love produces every day.

Watch programs on television that are about miracles. Don't watch violent, cruel, anger-filled shows that shrink your heart. Instead, record programs about joy, angels and miracles to uplift your soul and remind you that miracles do happen every day.

Put on your miracle glasses today! See everything through those glasses, and just before you go to sleep every night, review your day to see the hidden work of your angels. Examine anything that caused you frustration, delayed you or upset you, and try to imagine how it was a gift.

You may be surprised. I know that since I started doing this, I no longer see airport delays or cancellations as a frustrating inconvenience.

I am grateful for the work of my angels who know more than I do and are making sure that I am where I need to be. Who knows? I might meet someone important for my life on the next plane, or I may have missed an accident or a worse delay somewhere else.

Our guardian angels help us and guide us all the time. We need to learn to listen carefully, hear them and heed their advice! What we comprehend is so limited compared to the wisdom of the spiritual worlds. Be open. Listen carefully. Be grateful.

Miracles DO happen every day. Look for and rejoice in them!

MONDAY: CHOOSE YOUR MOODS

"The best way to cheer yourself up is to cheer someone else up."

—Mark Twain

Have you ever noticed how good it feels to make someone else laugh— or to cheer them up?

Today is the day you can develop your capacity to keep yourself joyful and spread that joy. No matter how you feel, how you woke up or what happens to you, your mission today is to *choose* to stay cheerful and share that mood!

Sustain that attitude of cheerfulness all day. Let nothing change it for more than a few moments. When something happens, like a person asking you to do something you don't want to do, cheerfully take the task on! Find the will forces to make sure that nothing can pull you out of your state of cheerfulness.

Find a way to feel good about everything that you do today and sustain the mood all day long, until the moment your head hits the pillow. At that moment, review the day and see how much better it flowed— and what miracles occurred.

Have you ever seen a sign outside a pub or bar that says "attitude-adjustment hour"? Perhaps each hour today can be a "cheerfulness-adjustment hour."

Keep track of what emotions creep in, and whenever the feeling of cheerfulness fades, immediately have a cheerfulness-adjustment moment! Think of all the reasons for being cheerful in your life, and if you can't think of any, just *choose* to be cheerful and see how your life changes!

Choose to be someone who will see the cup half full and not complain that it is half empty. Did you know that optimists live longer than pessimists? And cynical people may be harming their hearts? People who are cynical, stressed and distrustful have more inflammation in their bodies than others, and this leads to increased risks for cardio-vascular disease.

So now there are even more reasons to choose to be cheerful! You'll live longer, and more importantly, everyone will want you to!

TUESDAY: FACE ALL YOUR DIFFICULTIES WITH CHEERFULNESS

> "How do you go from where you are to where you want to be? I think you have to have enthusiasm for life."
>
> —Jim Valvano

Today's journey is to face *every* difficulty with cheerfulness and enthusiasm for the spiritual-growth experience it is!

When something goes wrong, instead of groaning, sighing and thinking, "Here we go again!" say to yourself, "Goodie!" or something like that! And then say, "I wonder what I am meant to be learning here?" Then proceed to look enthusiastically for that lesson.

Have you ever heard the story of two little boys at Christmas time—one a pessimist and one an optimist? They woke up Christmas morning and raced downstairs to see what gifts Santa had brought them. The pessimist saw a large pile of horse manure and was immediately disgusted. He muttered, "I *knew* I wasn't going to find anything good" and walked off unhappy.

The little optimist ran down the stairs, saw the manure and excitedly and enthusiastically started diving through it. When his parents asked him what he was doing, he said, "With all this horse manure, there has to be a horse somewhere!"

These two chose completely different responses to the same situation. We all have that choice—we can choose how to respond (and not react) to all situations. It may not be easy but we *can* do it! Practicing that discipline is a great way to develop our will.

We can say this prayer every night just before we go to sleep to keep us on the right path: *Heavenly Father, I pray that I did everything you wanted me to do today. If I didn't, give me the strength that I might do it tomorrow.*

Perhaps each night you work on cheerful enthusiasm (or anything else), you could say, "Tomorrow I shall have reached my goal of facing every difficulty with cheerful enthusiasm."

You will be amazed at how many less difficulties you encounter!

WEDNESDAY: BE PASSIONATE ABOUT BEING ENTHUSIASTIC

"I consider my ability to arouse enthusiasm among men the greatest asset I possess. The way to develop the best that is in a man is by appreciation and encouragement."

—Charles M. Schwab

Your goal for today is to be *passionate* about doing everything you do with enthusiasm—even if it is just washing dishes!

Appreciate and encourage other people with that same gusto. If you have a million little things to do, try to make each one, no matter how mundane, fun!

Mary, my great friend, has mastered that skill. She even tries to make her children's homework fun. It's much easier to be enthusiastic about something you enjoy doing, so whatever you do, find a way to make it fun.

Remember the story I told you earlier about Dianne, my friend in Australia?

In 2007, she was diagnosed with a tumor on her pituitary gland and was losing her vision and her speech. As you can imagine, it was a very stressful time. She called me, and despite her circumstances, she was still able to laugh.

She had and still has the most optimistic and cheerful attitude. She passionately embraced all the natural therapies with such enthusiasm and gusto that her condition vastly improved and she surprised her doctors with her progress. She could feel it herself and she did a tremendous amount of work to heal herself. A devout Christian, she had complete faith that she would be healed, but she did not passively wait for it to occur. She remained cheerful and diligently and passionately did her part of the healing. It worked!

If you are struggling to be enthusiastic and cheerful because you have a tough day ahead or a day full of chores, find gratitude in your heart and be enthusiastic that you are healthy enough to do the chores or tackle the day!

And if you do have a medical or other condition that is filling you with fear, breathe deeply. Challenge your thinking and handle it like Dianne or Jeni did. Research, find the right people to help you, take charge of your health, and enthusiastically do what you need to do to assist God in the healing process. Keep your heart full of faith and hope.

The Bible tells us seven times to "be of good cheer" in the face of all adversity. It does not say be of good cheer only during the good times!

God is always with you. Find peace in that. Have courage knowing you are not alone. And even if you don't believe in the Bible, it's still great advice. You can be disappointed and walk away from the pile of manure or you can passionately look for the gift hidden in it!

Your choice! *Your* will forces! *Your* life!

THURSDAY: SMILE ALL DAY—AT EVERYONE!

"Enthusiasm is contagious. Start an epidemic."

—Anonymous

Today, wake up and immediately smile! Before you climb out of bed, know that you are not alone, spiritually. The Divine is with you! Smile and say, "Good morning!" to those realms and to people! Smile with your heart and not just your face.

Smile at your family over breakfast, and when they ask you why you are smiling, tell them, "I have just decided to be cheerful today because I can!"

If you have chosen to smile from your heart at everyone today, you have chosen to be a spirit igniter! You will be spreading light, love and joy wherever you go. If you see a stranger on the street and smile, watch them smile back. If they don't, send them love, for they may not be used to people smiling at them or they may not know how to receive a gift with grace, because most people do not give love or joy freely.

Receive smiles from others today—especially babies and toddlers—and then smile back with both your face and your heart. It is a joyous exchange.

Have you ever walked into a house and had a child's eyes light up as he or she sees you? Or seen them run toward you shouting your name with excited, enthusiastic, unbridled joy? I am blessed because although I have not had children, my nephew and niece, Thomas and Clelia, did this to me when they were toddlers. Each time it happened, I thought my heart would burst with joy. I can't begin to explain the incredible feeling but I can recall it anytime I like and smile! If you have never had this happen, rent a child as quickly as possible! This is a feeling everyone should have at least once.

Imagine helping others to feel that level of joy from the way you greet them! Today is your chance. Go forth and make people's spirits sparkle!

FRIDAY: ALWAYS THINK WITH A JOYFUL HEART THAT THINGS WILL STEADILY IMPROVE

"We act as though comfort and luxury were the chief
requirements of life, when all that we need to make us really happy
is something to be enthusiastic about."

—Charles Kingsley

Remember, it is always sunny above the clouds! So no matter what challenges you face today or what problems you have, today is the day to make your heart joyful. Have absolute faith and believe that things will improve—maybe not in your preferred time frame, but in God's, which I'm sure will bring better results!

Who knows what a mess we would be in if we had always been given everything we thought we wanted, exactly when we wanted it! With the benefit of hindsight—how many of those things you wished for would have gone on to be a problem if your wishes were granted?

How many times have you had some past love that you thought you could not live without or some relationship that devastated you when it ended? Or maybe it was a job you didn't get or business you thought you wanted that fell through? Although you were disappointed at the time or even devastated, when you look back now, you probably realize it was the best thing that could have happened to you.

For me, one of those situations was when I was 45, losing all the money I had made. I was half a million dollars in debt! I must say, had I known about cheerful enthusiasm at that time, my will forces would have been a lot stronger by now!

But in retrospect, this experience was one of the best things that ever happened to me. Not only did I finally understand in every cell of my body that money did *not* bring security, but the loss also brought me to the u.s. Without being in this gracious and generous country with incredible, amazing teachers who have blessed me and continue to bless me, I would not have found financial stability as quickly nor the spiritual path I am meant to be on.

Today is your day to reflect on how your life's "disasters" turned into blessings—or at least on how something good came out of something horrible or not so good. God has a way of doing that! He does not create the horrible events, but He does work to turn them into good somehow.

There is always sunshine above the clouds. Know that. Believe it with every cell in your body. Do your work. Wait patiently while doing your work, with a joyful heart full of certainty *or faith* that the clouds will pass and the sun will shine again.

SATURDAY: **FIND YOUR WORK**

"When a person applies enthusiasm to his job, the job will itself
become alive with exciting new possibilities."

—Norman Vincent Peale

Your job is your job, but it can also be your work, depending on how
you look at it and how you do it. Your *work* is manna for the soul. It
fulfills you and satisfies you, and it usually involves serving others.

Go to your job today and *make it* your work. *Everyone* in every job
serves others in some way—the boss, colleagues, customers or clients,
the country or the community. It does not matter how lowly you feel
your job is, you are part of a serving team. Teams only function well
when *all* parts do their best to work with and serve all the others.

Author and inventor Buckminster Fuller said, "The whole is greater
than the sum of the parts." That means that when we all connect and
contribute to the team, the results are much better.

Ambitious, selfish people who ignore, harm or cut down others for
their own personal goals may realize apparent short-term success, but
their success will probably not last and they will not be happy, fulfilled
or satisfied.

They will not be honored because they are not honoring others.
People who think, "My pie will be smaller if you have some of it!" don't
understand the laws of life! Giving more, helping more and serving
more can only bring you more—although that should not be your
motivation, of course!

Your motivation is to serve others, and when you focus on that, you
may be surprised at how joy, contentment, fulfillment, satisfaction and
financial rewards appear in your life. They just magically flow in while
you are focused on others.

If you know in your heart that the job you are in is not for you,
complete your tasks and do the job the best you can while you look for
your *real* work. This will make your job less arduous and may miraculously lead you to your real work.

Never grumble again about your job! For starters, you have one—millions don't. Be grateful! You also have the choice to make your job enjoyable, even if it is making beds in a motel while there is a football team in the room making suggestive comments about you! Yes—this happened to me. And although it was not the most pleasant experience, I smiled and laughed as I told them I would come back later—when they had gone!

The more you grumble and complain, the less people want to be around you and the more you attract other grumbling, complaining spirit phoofers. You are creating your own special set of storm clouds. You are not contributing to the team—in fact, you may be aiding in destroying it. Never underestimate the power of one spirit phoofer on a whole organization. If that is you, stop it today!

Banish any negative thoughts about your job. Enthusiastically find good things instead. Become a spirit igniter. Serve others the best you can, and find your true work. It may be right under your nose!

CHAPTER 12

A WEEK OF EQUANIMITY

"Be still and know that I AM."

—Psalms 46:10

YOUR SEVEN MINUTES

What does "equanimity" mean to you? Are you saying to yourself that you can't even spell it, let alone know what it is?

Is your nervous system almost always on red alert? Do you panic, feel stressed or worry a lot? Do you see life as a series of crises? Why?

Do you find it hard to let go of "stuff" that has happened to you? Do you take time each day to seek God's peace?

What creates a deep foundation of peace or calm in you—not a passive state, but one in which you are aware and alert, yet relaxed and alive?

Have you ever felt a state of inner peace and contentment? Enter into that memory, and identify the aspects that brought you peace.

AMANDA'S TAKE ON EQUANIMITY

"Rejoice in the Lord always! Again I will say, Rejoice! Let your gentleness be known to all men. The Lord is at hand. In nothing be anxious, but in everything, by prayer and petition with thanksgiving, let your requests be made known to God. And the peace of God, which surpasses all understanding, will guard your hearts and your thoughts in Christ Jesus."

—Philippians 4:6-7

Equanimity is that state of composure which the Bible speaks of as *the peace that passeth understanding*. It refers to someone who is perfectly composed in even the most adverse situation, and it comes from divine inspiration.

In a state of equanimity, we are totally at peace, connected to brotherly love and composed, and always seem to know the right thing to do. We can see the whole and put ourselves into another person's shoes and yet also hold firm to what needs to be done.

Equanimity results in brotherly love, courage and other great qualities. Many see equanimity as a divine gift, and it can be seen clearly at times of crisis when composure seems to "descend" on a person.

If you can work towards equanimity and live within it most of the time, your life will be joyful beyond measure!

PERFECT EQUANIMITY
Look how a mirror
will reflect with perfect equanimity
all actions
before
it

There is no act in this world
that will ever cause the mirror to look away.
There is no act in this world that will
Ever make the mirror
Say "no."

The mirror, like perfect love, will just keep giving
of itself to all
before
it.

How did the mirror get like that, so polite,
so grand, so compassionate?

It watched God.

Yes, the mirror remembers the Beloved
looking into itself as the Beloved shaped existence's heart
and the mirror's
Soul.[1]

—Daniel Ladinsky

Many definitions I've encountered describe equanimity mostly as a state of mind. The heart-and-soul aspect I really found useful was from Robert Sardello in his wonderful book *The Power of Soul: Living the Twelve Virtues* (Hampton Roads Publishing Company, 2003. Reprinted with permission):

"Suppression of an emotion can outwardly look like equanimity. Equanimity does not look flat, for it is not an absence. The person of equanimity bears a countenance of buoyancy, accompanied with an inner light that shines from the soul, lighting the eyes expressed as an engaged interest in all that one encounters. Equanimity concerns balancing the relationship among emotions, thought and will."

Another interesting definition came from a talk given by a Buddhist teacher named Gil Fronsdal (www.insightmeditationcenter.org), who kindly gave me permission to reproduce it here:

"The English word 'equanimity' translates two separate Pali words used by the Buddha. Each represents a different aspect of equanimity. 'Upekkha,' meaning 'to look over,' refers to the equanimity that arises from the power of observation, the ability to see without being caught by what we see . . . to see with patience. We might understand this as 'seeing with understanding.'

"The second word often translated as 'equanimity' is 'tatramajjhattata,' meaning 'to stand in the middle of all this.'"

I wondered if this meant that we are in a state of equanimity when we are in a balanced place and can clearly see from a higher perspective and really understand what is going on at all levels—to be involved and at the same time observing?

When the concept of equanimity came to me as one of the practices for this book, I thought, "What do I know about equanimity?" It's something I have always wanted and can never seem to achieve!

As a young girl I wanted to be serene. (If you know me, you're laughing out loud at this!) In my twenties I decided that what I really wanted to be was "bubbling serene"—so that I was not boring! (You are probably laughing louder now!)

I suspect the inspiration that came to me about being "bubbling serene" was an indicator that we can feel peace and yet be alive, interested, enthusiastic, active and dynamically participating in what we are meant to be doing in life, all the while sensing the bigger picture of what really is going on—that all will be well no matter how it looks now.

Years later, when I was a convener of a conference on ergonomics, I was driving one of our speakers around Sydney. He asked me, "What is the thing you want most in life?" This, at the time, was not in my normal range of topics for conversation, and to my complete surprise, out of my mouth fell the words "inner peace." Honestly, I looked around and thought, "Who said that?"

I didn't really think about it much after that. It was just part of me that submerged back into the chaos of daily life—until . . . I started writing this book. And then I did some big-time thinking, meditation and reflection on equanimity! And I realized that what came out of my mouth that day had been a true desire; a reminder for me to pay attention to how I could develop inner peace. (Apparently, I'm no closer to it than when I was a little girl! But I am changing that after doing this research and writing this book! I hope reading it has the same effect on you.)

When we can hold the big picture and remember God is in charge of everything, that most things happen for a reason and we always have more help than we can imagine, we keep our sense of inner peace. Our free will can interfere with our planned progress—so staying connected to God and recognizing the spiritual design for our lives is essential.

Maybe equanimity is just a fancy word for being conscious of how everything interacts, seeing the bigger picture always and having inner peace at all times, in all situations, no matter what happens!

I have a feeling that equanimity was the last chapter in this book because it is a blend of the concepts of all the other chapters.

ENEMIES OF INNER PEACE

ENEMY #1:

NOT LETTING GO—OR LETTING GO TOO MUCH!

Not letting go of past hurts and wounds, old stuff, expectations, a desire for our own outcomes, judgment, selfishness, greed, desperation and other neediness can destroy our peace.

We find ourselves feeling victimized, needing to be right, fearful, unforgiving, needing to control and on and on! Most of us need to let go of *at least* one thing. *You* know what you must let go of so you can be free to move on. Make the choice to do it now.

Here is a fun way of looking at letting go:

Imagine you have a sack of potatoes on one side of you and an empty sack on the other. You are going to pull out a potato for *every* person who has ever offended you, wounded you, upset you, harmed you or "done" anything wrong to you in your eyes. Write their name on the potato, place it in the empty sack, and continue doing this until you have covered every single person. Then start on the situations in life that were "unfair" or not right or whatever it is that you judged should not have happened. Write on a potato for each one of them.

When you have finished, pick up the newly filled sack of potatoes and carry that with you everywhere you go, every day, for the rest of your life. Take it to bed, work, church, parties, social events, the bathroom, sporting or community events—*everywhere* you go.

After six weeks, what will those potatoes be like? Yessirree! They will be turning to liquid, moldy, filled with fungus, nasty-smelling and just generally be horrible. Yet that is similar to what you are carrying around inside you!

All those hurts, resentments, anger, fears and patterns of the past sit inside you and rot away your soul.

YOU HAVE TO DROP YOUR POTATOES!

Forgive and move on. Those potatoes are taking up the space that light, hope and joy are meant to occupy. Do you really want moldy potatoes instead of light, hope and joy? It's your choice!

Life is full of lessons to learn, unlearn and relearn, and the future is too full of exciting possibilities for us to waste our time focusing on those rotten potatoes.

Carefully examine your thoughts. They can keep alive old, negative stuff and destructive emotions and patterns. Your heart is wiser and wastes no time on the bitterness and disappointments generated by feeling a victim and having expectations or desires for your *own* outcomes.

We need to seek God's help and take responsibility for ourselves and for what we have created. Find all the judgments, selfishness, greed, neediness, fears and anything else you are hanging onto and let them go. DROP THOSE POTATOES, TOO!

Letting go of these things frees you up, makes you lighter and allows you to see or sense wonderful things that may be coming towards you from the future.

ENEMY #2:

INDIFFERENCE

If you let go so much that you become indifferent or just don't care for others or the effect you have on them, there is no "brotherly love." There is just self-centeredness and isolation.

To be indifferent is to "go to sleep" and separate ourselves. Separation is the opposite of equanimity. Separation robs us of equanimity. With indifference, we withdraw from God, people and life, and disconnect from the lessons available to us.

Indifference can be felt as a sort of numbness or maybe a passive-aggressiveness that we allow to overtake us. "*WhatEVER!*" is an expression that is common, but what does that mean anyway? The tone of voice in which it is usually expressed is derogatory and often accompanied by someone walking away disrespectfully, leaving everyone frustrated, hurt or angry. Or it can be said in the flat tone that indicates no life—that there is no life force behind the words, and that the person has given up, separated, withdrawn or retreated into no feeling.

Indifference can kill your soul! Everything you do, say and think has an impact on someone else *and* the world. You are not an island! You are, whether you accept it or not, intricately connected to everyone else and to the spiritual realms, so be considerate and conscious of your connections. Be aware of others around you. You are affecting them and they are affecting you.

A simple example of this can be seen in planes. Have you ever been trying to board when the plane is running late? The flight attendants are constantly asking people to allow others to pass by, and yet, there are always those unconscious, indifferent souls who spend five minutes organizing themselves while there are 200 people lined up behind them, waiting.

That person holding up all the others is not in a state of equanimity. *They* may be calm, but they are unaware of the distress or frustration they are causing. They are indifferent and either don't care or are not aware that they are inconveniencing many others.

Equanimity does not mean finding peace by being indifferent, separated, calm, bland or flatlining all emotions! It is a very active state. We can feel our emotions but hopefully balance them with an understanding of the bigger scheme of things, which brings a sense of peace.

From that state of wisdom, we feel brotherly love and compassion and view things as they really are—not as we *perceive* them to be. We may feel very strongly about something, but we are careful not to impose our ideas on others. We allow them the freedom to make their own decisions and choices, no matter how hard that is to watch.

If we cling to the idea that others must do something because *we* think it is best for them, we are taking *their* free will away and imposing ours on them. It is frustrating and disappointing for everyone.

So rather than becoming indifferent to (or separated from) what others do as a way to avoid our *own* disappointment, we need to accept that they are responsible for their own lives, directions and outcomes. We remain in a relationship with them and are still involved, but perhaps more in a supportive role, with patience and grace.

ENEMY #3:

RUSHING, WORRY AND STRESS

Being caught in hurrying, worrying and stress is another way to destroy equanimity through separation. These states all arise from our thoughts or judgments, and would not appear if we remained connected to God and others.

RUSHING

It took me a long time, but one day it dawned on me (in a blinding flash of the obvious!) that one of the major things that disturbed my peace was rushing. Rushing is not the same as moving quickly! Some people can move quickly yet also remain conscious of the whole. We can achieve a lot during the day by moving quickly with-out rushing or feeling rushed.

The minute I start to rush, I disconnect and focus solely on the panic rapidly rising in me that I will not be ready on time, or be at the place I need to be, or make an appointment on time—or whatever it might be.

Realizing that rushing was an issue for me was a great learning experience. From that day on, I have made sure that I am organized, and the likelihood of last-minute changes or rushing is minimal. Life is much smoother and more pleasant.

I now try to catch myself as soon as the state of rushing sneaks up on me. I take a deep breath and stop it! I change what I am saying to myself. I drop to my heart, relax and find that the old adage "more haste, less speed" is really true!

What does rushing do to you?

WORRY

There is a difference between worry and concern. When we worry, we either can't do anything about the situation or don't do anything about it. We allow our thoughts to run round and round, creating a cycle of stress and distress.

Concern is knowing there's a problem and taking care of it, or doing what we can do and letting it go, or just being conscious that the problem is there. Worry is counterproductive and disturbs equanimity. Concern is not distressing; it simply makes us aware and sensibly cautious.

Did you know that Olympic and elite athletes spend about three hours a day mentally rehearsing? They not only train physically, they also train mentally by meditating and repeatedly imagining themselves performing perfectly. They shoot perfect baskets or hurdle brilliantly or make perfect maneuvers time after time in their minds.

As they do this, micro muscle movements occur and they unconsciously train their bodies physically to make perfect moves. Vividly imagining what they *want to have happen*—with sound, movement and feeling—facilitates their success.

Think about worry for a moment—what is it? Worry is vividly imagining what you DON'T *want to have happen*—usually in Technicolor, with surround sound! It is accompanied with all the feelings, horror and fears that you would have if the thing you are worrying about were actually happening!

If we know that *vividly imagining* what you DO want to have happen makes that significantly more likely to occur, why would we think that vividly imagining what we DON'T want to have happen is okay? Worry, in my opinion, is not only useless and a waste of time, but it may well be harmful!

It is very useful to be aware of what you say to yourself and have an alternative series of optimistic thoughts to replace the stress creating thoughts of worry. Make a list of things you would rather program into your imagination and repeat them often.

If you are worried about exams, tests, interviews or a meeting, *do* the work you are supposed to do and prepare appropriately instead of trapping yourself in negative, worrying thoughts and inaction.

Repeat (this takes an act of will) preferred sentences like, "I am well-prepared," "I have done the work. I will be breathing and calm," "I am full of trust and faith that if I am meant to be in this job, I will" or the many other statements you could make relevant to your situation. It's simple and easy to make these positive statements, and it's amazing how *few* people are aware of their destructive "criticizer" thoughts.

Move to your heart, where the wisdom lives. Your heart will guide you, tell you what you need to do at that time, settle you down, put things in perspective and bring equanimity.

STRESS

Sometimes we have to push ourselves to do things—which we can perceive as stressful. But if we push ourselves and achieve a lot, we usually feel good at the end of the day. It may have been exhausting, but we feel we were productive. If we allow feelings of stress to take over, however, we paralyze ourselves and don't do anything.

If someone says, "Don't stress about that," it doesn't mean, "Don't do anything." Instead, it probably means *do something* but stop stressing about it!

Remember, stress is a *fact* of life; it doesn't have to be a *way* of life!

The interesting thing about stress is that there can be situations that create physical stress, such as extreme cold, heat or poor health, but we rarely mean that when we say "stress."

It's more common to use the word "stress" when we mean anxiety or tension. We say we are "stressed" when we are anxious, fearful or out of balance—it's a *psychological* state that causes a *physiological* reaction. In terms of psychology, there are no events, people or things that stress us! It is what *we tell ourselves or imagine* about the event that occurred that causes the stress.

For example, imagine four women sitting in a house on a hill. They see a thunderstorm approaching. One woman loves thunderstorms and she is excited and can't wait for it to arrive. Her body releases pleasurable hormones and chemicals.

Another woman is indifferent to thunderstorms, and her body chemistry stays the same.

The third woman is terrified of thunderstorms because one frightened her when she was a little girl. When she sees the storm, she panics and is filled with anxiety and fear. Her body is swarming with nasty stress hormones that make her feel terrible.

The fourth woman is concerned by the thunderstorm but knows to take certain precautions and prepares wisely. She does what needs to be done and might push herself to do it, but all without stress.

Such different responses to exactly the same event! Can you see how our old brain can control us if we are not conscious of what is going on? We lose touch with reality. Instead, *what we perceive, say to ourselves and expect to happen* rules us.

If we perceive a storm as dangerous and scary, it *will* be! Others may see it as God putting on a fireworks display! If it really is a dangerous storm, a cautious, prudent person will review the situation, prepare and flow with the requirements. Monitor your perceptions and thoughts and challenge the ones that cause stress and inaction.

When we allow stress to rule our lives, we have little chance of finding equanimity.

ENEMY #4:

EXTREME EMOTION

There is a huge difference between negative emotions and intuition or "gut feelings." Reflect for a minute on the difference between an acute emotion like panic (which I feel in my chest) and a gut feeling.

Acute panic "attacks" us! Before we know it, we have stopped breathing and can only see our own perceived or real "danger"—we are totally unaware of anything else.

On the other hand, a "gut feeling" is more a quiet voice warning us that something somewhere is not right (or something is right!). It creates an awareness or a conscious state in us, putting us on alert so we are not blindsided and can take appropriate action.

Extreme emotional states break down conditions that facilitate equanimity. While I was meditating on this chapter, this wonderful image came to me:

Negative emotions are like horses that gallop in, unseen or unnoticed by us, and somehow, these horses put us on their backs and ride away at high speed! We are miles down the road, completely focused on hanging onto the wildly galloping horse, before we even know where we are!

When we are in the state of equanimity, we *see* the "horse" and *feel* the emotion, but we choose not to be swept up and carried away on the galloping horse. We recognize we have a choice. We can be conscious of what is *really* happening and make wiser decisions.

If we are in a position to observe what is happening, rather than unknowingly being carried away with the horses of emotion, then we can take a deep breath, "step outside" ourselves, review the situation as it *really* is, and then step back in and participate in an appropriate way that brings peace, harmony or balance.

It would probably be a fun exercise to start talking about the horses of emotion in your family—make it a routine dinner table discussion! "What horse of emotion carried you off today?"

ENEMY #5:

REACTING RATHER THAN FEELING

Feelings are those inner "knowings" or "gut feelings" we have all had at some time in our lives. Those situations where we could say, "I just knew it!" and we most likely did! The heart is far more powerful than most of us imagine.

If we can learn to place our attention in our hearts and stay there for a while before our negative emotions send us off on another horse of reaction, if we can see with the "eyes" of our heart, then every aspect of our lives will change.

The heart can be (if we are conscious) the balance point between our emotions and everything else that is happening—both in the cosmos and the rest of our world! It can give you insights and wisdom and can guide you through the "feeling language" it uses so you can respond rather than react.

We have to listen carefully for the guidance from our hearts and those gut feelings. They can be easily missed in the chaos of daily life—and certainly when that emotional horse is about to, or has, run away with us!

ENEMY #6:

DOUBT AND FEAR

> "There is nothing more dreadful than the habit of doubt. Doubt separates people. It is a poison that disintegrates friendships and breaks up pleasant relations. It is a thorn that irritates and hurts; it is a sword that kills.
>
> —Buddha

> "Doubt makes the mountain which faith can move."
>
> —Proverb

The English word *doubt* is derived from the Latin word *duo*, meaning "two." *Double* originated from the same word as *doubt*. To doubt means to be "double-minded."

The two quotes above demonstrate in part the double nature of doubt. It can be useful or harmful. There is a big difference between the *habit* of doubting and recognizing doubt as an intermittent warning sign.

If we are in the habit of never believing anything we hear or see, we are doomed to a life of rigidity, ignorance, fear, denial and suspicion. If we unquestioningly believe everything we hear or learn, we are in danger of being led astray by doctrines that are false and potentially harmful, or overwhelmed by all the opposing conditions and information we discover. And if we sit in the middle and never have the courage to make a choice, we are doomed to a life of indecision and procrastination!

If we imagine a line with doubt at one end and its opposite, certainty, at the other, the pivot point in the middle would be faith that comes through the wisdom of the heart.

Doubt is a part of life, and I believe it's often an invitation to explore further rather than continue on a particular path. Certainty about everything blocks learning as much as disbelieving everything does. Neither provides the balanced view of wisdom.

I, and many friends of mine, have gone through our greatest growth periods after doubt crept—or swept!—into our daily life! The doubts may have been about our purpose in life or the wisdom of a relationship or choice. They may have been about our chosen career or some other major life activity.

Perhaps fear and doubt live in the gut! When we have a gut feeling that something is wrong, perhaps it's a sign we don't have enough information for clear thinking. Our guts cannot digest and make sense of what is going on. Perceive doubts as an invitation to seek more information, instead of ignoring, being paralyzed by or sneering at them. The information you uncover may help you grow and develop as a spiritual human being.

If we just stew in doubt and walk around thinking and feeling, "I don't know!" "What if it isn't?" or "What if it is?" we do not use courage or our will forces to act on the signal that we need more information. This is a major reason for procrastination—rightly so in some cases. Action without adequate information may lead to unwise choices.

Often our gut feelings are trying to warn us about something we are contemplating doing or being involved in, whether that is a relationship, a business venture or a life change. The way we "hear" that warning is doubt.

It's interesting that when asked, many famous business leaders say they made their best decisions by "following my gut feeling."

How many times have you felt uneasy, doubtful or uncertain about making a commitment to someone—personally or in business? If we ignore that warning and try to rationalize or intellectualize the decision, we don't feel peace, even though the facts *seem* logical and sensible. Your insides are screaming out at you, "Don't do this!" through the vehicle of doubt!

Walking down the aisle for my first marriage, I knew I was doing the wrong thing. *I knew it.* But I did not have the courage to stop the ceremony. I had doubts well before that day but did not act on them.

Can you recall doing something you just knew was the wrong thing to do, yet you still did it and it turned out a disaster? That can be the consequence of doubt ignored or unexplored!

FAITH AND TRUST

Doubt that denies, rejects, questions or blocks faith in God and the wisdom of nature and the spiritual world is, in my opinion, a path to unconsciousness, hopelessness, stagnation, pain and misery. It's not really doubt—it's cynicism or skepticism.

Trusting, having faith, hearing our inner wisdom and living spiritually are critical for equanimity. We can have composure on our own, but true, deep, abiding equanimity, the peace that passes all understanding, comes from God or the Holy Spirit.

Brenda, our wonderful next-door neighbor in Vermont, told me a story that epitomizes deep equanimity from God. Two of her nephews were riding their trail bikes on her father's property. They had a head-on crash in which one of them was critically injured. He was not breathing when found, had skull fractures, facial fractures and a compound fractured femur, and his right leg was almost severed above the knee.

While waiting for the medical helicopter, Brenda was extremely upset, and as she was comforting the sisters of one of the boys, "out of the blue" she heard God's voice say very clearly, "Both boys are going to be fine." Immediately she was filled with an incredible sense of peace and *knew* they would recover. She didn't know *how* it would happen, because the injuries were so bad, but she had absolute faith it *would* happen.

In intensive care, the family was told that the boy, because of the severity of his injuries and the time he would be in intensive care, *would* develop infections, pneumonia and blood clots. None of those things happened. He had an extraordinary, rapid recovery and surprised everyone. Instead of it taking a year for him to get back to normal activities, it took four months! That's the power of God in action—He makes good out of terrible things, and Brenda's faith and trust helped that happen.

Fear (the opposite of faith) disrupts everything and prevents inner peace. If Brenda, a nurse, had chosen to fear what was going to happen based on her past experiences in hospitals, her faith would have wavered. Instead, she *chose* to believe what God said, although she knew the injuries were life-threatening.

How we choose to deal with the past or the future is the source of many fears. We can look backward or forward, anticipating a repeat of a terrible pattern or something worse, or we can choose to trust the wisdom of the spiritual worlds and do our part by listening, praying and holding faith as Brenda did.

We don't like change, even though change is one of the only constants in the world. We fear change because we don't *know* what will happen and we don't like uncertainty. Fear hinders or prevents faith and the development of the capacity for equanimity. Fear can paralyze us and it stops our life forces flowing. When we let fear over-take our faith, we are killing ourselves!

Faith overcomes fear. Make a choice: Will you operate today from fear, or faith and trust?

Here is a meditation that may help you actually *feel* the presence of equanimity and understand it a bit better.

MEDITATION FOR COURAGE

"We must eradicate from the soul all fear and terror of what comes towards us from the future.

We must look forward with absolute equanimity to whatever comes, and we must think only that whatever comes is given to us by a world direction full of wisdom.

It is part of what we must learn during this age, namely to act out of pure trust in the ever present help of the spiritual world; truly nothing else will do if our courage is not to fail us.

Therefore let us discipline our will and let us seek the awakening from within ourselves, every morning and every evening."[2]

—Rudolf Steiner

ENEMY #7:

THE CYCLES

Another friend of mine went into paralysis and fear when she started doubting her chosen career. She was in a great job, the company loved her work, and she was very successful, yet she was plagued by doubts about her career choice. That expanded into doubt, or negative emotions about who *she* was, and what she wanted to do with her life.

Her gut sent her signals—gut feelings interpreted as doubt—that she was not meant to be in the profession she had chosen. But instead of exploring that and all the consequences with equanimity (i.e., through her heart), her doubts took control! She was comparing herself with what she perceived to be more experienced, professional peers, and others in her personal life. This led to a cycle of negative thoughts but not action. She found herself depressed, anxious and unhappy.

We can be conscious of doubt and then freeze into fear rather than exploring the cause or source of the doubt. Of course, when this is happening to you, it's not at all obvious! You just feel enormously stuck, worried, depressed, disturbed or stressed. You don't even realize that you have tapes playing the same negative, fear-inspiring junk over and over! You have to stop the cycle!

It takes an act of will—*will power*—to do this. We have to make a decision to stop the negative thought cycle and tap into our hearts. Be conscious that a horse of fear and anxiety has run away with you. See the horse for what it is, and make conscious decisions to listen to God.

Confusion takes over when we are not in the flow, often because we are not doing what we are supposed to or we don't have enough information.

The minute we are aware that we are trapped within our self-talk (which usually is when we are carried away with fear, depression or anxiety)—we must DO SOMETHING! Go for a run or exercise (after checking with a doctor!) until you are so absorbed that you can't *think* anymore. Listen to uplifting music or read uplifting books or meditate. Do some housework, or best of all, volunteer to visit a hospital, church, orphanage or shelter and be of service.

When we do things prayerfully, or as a service, we often do feel better because it takes our minds off ourselves. That lets us put our needs in proper perspective.

When you are in your heart, being of service, perhaps the truth about what is going on will emerge. You will have a sense of equanimity gently flow through you—often without even knowing it. At the end of the time of serving others, your soul is lighter, a miracle has happened, *you* feel better and you have a sense of what will help *your* situation. By now, you know miracles happen in the heart all the time!

I think it should be compulsory for everyone to work in some form of service to others for a few days every year! If you go home consumed by all your own problems and don't feel joyful for the blessings in your life, including all the struggles, doubts, difficulties and the fact that you *have* a life, spend more time in service! Working in hospitals helped me learn that lesson early in my career. It was a real blessing and helped me develop empathy.

Once we realize there *are* messages from our hearts and guts and we listen for them, we need to act on them. Have the courage to explore the questions that are arising from that doubt, and have more courage to accept the answers.

Doubt can be a doorway to inner peace and wisdom—seek that doorway!

ENEMY #8:
SELFISHNESS

> "The great danger for family life, in the midst of any society whose idols are pleasure, comfort and independence, lies in the fact that people close their hearts and become selfish."
>
> —Pope John Paul II

Extremely selfish people have a sense of themselves *only*—or worse, they have a very good sense of others and how to manipulate the situation to achieve their own goals. Selfishness leads to separation, either from others or God.

On the other hand, people who exist as if they don't matter are separated from themselves and therefore separated from God and others. To find the balance, we need to develop a true sense of ourselves and a sense of community—to recognize that *we are always an integral part of a community, of the whole*. We are individuals and part of the whole at the same time. Losing sight of either one of those blocks our capacity for equanimity.

The critical factor here is *disregard* for others or *disregard* for the self. To have regard for someone means to respect or honor them, or see them with our heart, so selfishness or extreme self*less*ness are both all about dishonoring, disrespecting and closing our hearts "eyes and ears."

BROTHERLY LOVE

"The firm basis of all spiritual power is equanimity. Quietude is a very positive state; an active peace, contagious, powerful, which controls and calms, which puts everything in order, organizes.... True quietude is a very great force, a very great strength. Calmness belongs to the strong."[3]

—Sri Arubindo & the Mother

It came to me one morning that equanimity results in brotherly love. This made me wonder, "What does brotherly love mean?" I was not sure at all! Did you know that the Greek word for "brotherly love" is *philadelphia* and it's mentioned in Revelations in the Bible? I didn't! DUH!

John tells us in the Bible (John 4:12[4]) that if we love one another, God abides in us and His love is perfected. How we physically and emotionally treat others is basically how we are choosing to treat God. What are you choosing?

Brotherly love is present when we are finally conscious enough to see the *true* spiritual being in everyone we meet—our "brothers"—and that we *really are all one*. It's a pretty big concept!

And I can only imagine that if we make even teeny little steps in the direction of unconditional or brotherly love, we will be doing very well in our spiritual growth! Any movement away from judgment and towards truly seeing others in their magnificence, realizing that we all have God inside us, brings us closer to equanimity and real brotherly love.

HOW TO FIND EQUANIMITY?

Use your gifts
Observe, don't judge
See yourself as you really are
Filter everything through your pure heart
Have faith, trust and courage
Live in harmony with the rhythms of nature
Take responsibility for your own life—live with integrity
Be receptive and open to what is emerging
Be content and choose your feelings
Control desire and comparisons

MY FRIEND KATHY

My friend Kathy is a picture of equanimity and brotherly love. She is very wise, calm, patient, optimistic and encouraging; she is highly conscious, intuitive, spiritual and kind and sees the potential that can unfold in people. She nourishes the unfolding—in the *other* person's time frame! She still feels what most of us feel, but the horses of emotion never carry her away.

Being around Kathy is what I imagine a flower would feel like when it is planted in fertile soil—she *is* the fertile soil, rain and sunshine that allow the flower to blossom. And at the same time Kathy takes good care of, and makes some time for, herself. She rarely rushes and is never in a state of stressed chaos, despite having a million things to do. There is a sense of groundedness with her, and just having her in the room makes me feel calm and peaceful! Do you know anyone like that? Hang around them—a lot!

Kathy is a role model for us in this section. I have listed what we need to do and then how Kathy manifests it in everyday life. Pattern your lives in a similar manner and your life will flow with equanimity.

1. USE YOUR GIFTS

Aim to live in a state of understanding. Our work as humans is to work and grow spiritually and be actively using our gifts to fulfill our purpose in life and do what we are meant to be doing, while still contributing positively to *others*—even if that contribution is just to support others in what they do or to love them *despite* what they do or think. Identify and use the gifts you have been given to do these things.

WHAT WOULD KATHY DO?

Kathy is amazing in her insights and perceptions of her own gifts and the difficulties others face in their life path. One of these gifts is the ability to gently offer suggestions in the most subtle way to share an alternative approach or thought for us to look at if we choose. Her suggestions are usually very good at helping us see what we really are meant to be doing, yet she is not attached to our following her suggestion!

My husband Ken and Mary, my other mentor, are also brilliant at that! I, on the other hand, am very good at offering advice and trying to fix your life! You don't even have to ask for it! It's one of my gifts! If we see a need and try to help or fix things without being asked, it can be detrimental for others and/or our relationship. Our job is to listen for or recognize requests for assistance—direct or subtle.

Our opinions and advice are generally not what people want to hear, even if they are great ideas. The way I offer them is not so much as an invitation but as a strong suggestion! And yes, I have asked Kathy, Ken and Mary to coach me!

I am also learning to offer help with no attachment—and only when I am asked in some way! Instead of feeling I know what is best for others and expecting them to do it, I am working at letting go and giving freely, when asked. No strings!

And I'm working on fixing only me and doing what I am meant to be doing.

We are all works in progress—but I now realize I am in charge *only* of my *own progress! HA HA!*

2. OBSERVE, DON'T JUDGE

We must not judge others or break off our relationship with them if they don't do what we think is right or what we want them to do.

To love someone without judgment really does take an act of will—it's hard work for most of us. We are supposed to love them *no matter what they do or don't do.*

I can recall many situations in my life where everything would have been transformed if I had had the courage, capacity and will to love with *brotherly* love, to treat the other as a special, wise spiritual being, stay connected, and allow their own wisdom to unfold versus my fix for them!

WHAT WOULD KATHY DO?

Kathy's favorite saying is, "Observe, don't judge."

She observes, waits patiently for a feeling to unfold, "drops to her heart," senses what it tells her to do, and then responds—she does not react!

I, on the other hand, am often quick to process (not necessarily accurate but quick!), sum things up and decide a course of action, then I immediately embark on it. Only afterwards do I sometimes see the chaos I caused and drama I created! If I had been seeing through my heart like Kathy, I would have avoided a great deal of stress—for me and everyone else!

Imagine what it would be like if we had compassion for everyone and could give them grace, or at the very least understanding, rather than judgment?

3. SEE YOURSELF AS YOU REALLY ARE

If we can see and accept ourselves as we truly are, and we allow those around us the freedom to be who they really are, brotherly love flows. Larry Byram, founder of Higher Alignment (www.higheralignment. com), says once we can see ourselves clearly, we can stop projecting onto everyone else and see *them* as they really are!

What would life be like if we felt safe, secure and loved as *ourselves*! If we really understood who we are, we could free ourselves to focus on helping others see their own beauty. Larry Byram also says, "When we know our own goodness, we allow others to connect with theirs."

Who do you know, love and totally accept despite all that you know about them? How do you treat them? Can you treat others more like this? *Will* you?

WHAT WOULD KATHY DO?

Kathy would create a situation in which a person feels great about him- or herself. She already sees herself very clearly, knows herself well and feels good about what she sees! From that place of equanimity, she can find the real beauty in others, even if they can't see it themselves, and she can be gracious with them, because she can give herself grace.

Are you a "projector"? Do you routinely project your stuff onto others? Or do others feel good about themselves around you? Do you bring out the best in others? Do you help others to see the "astonishing light" that is inside them?

Now is a great time to start accepting yourself and people for who they are.

John Gottman, an expert on relationships who runs the "love lab" at Washington State University, says that the "paradox of relationships is that people change when they feel accepted for who they are." I would add to that: when they feel *loved* for who they are, despite their behaviors and beliefs.

4. FILTER EVERYTHING THROUGH YOUR PURE HEART

If we filtered everything through the wisdom of our hearts *before* we acted or spoke, our lives would be transformed. (Remember, the heart is the seat of equanimity.)

How do we do that? It's pretty simple: Make a conscious effort to place your attention, an issue or people *into* your heart and hold them there until you "hear" from your heart what to do or not do. Sometimes you do nothing but hold people in your heart and allow the heart to work its magic! It's not so easy, but it is very simple!

Our hearts are the connection between the spiritual worlds and us. The wisdom of the spiritual worlds can be perceived and understood by our hearts, so our pure heart will always receive the right answer! When we make judgments, we always have answers as well, only they are rarely the right ones!

Our job is to listen to and trust our heart for information about what is going on and what we need to do, and for it to tell us how we can behave or contribute. Interestingly, that behavior may be to cheerfully wait, with a good attitude, patience and equanimity, and be *confident* that something good will emerge!

WHAT WOULD KATHY DO?

As soon as Kathy hears something that is likely to, or starts to, trigger a reaction, she uses the "drop to your heart technique." I have been doing this consciously since the Sacred Service class, but to catch yourself in time, just before you are about to react, takes dedication and attention! It involves "hovering" above the situation for a fraction of a second, seeing what is going on, stopping, breathing, taking the issue to your heart, listening carefully for guidance and *then* responding—all in a couple of seconds!

When I can do it, it seems to work very well. The process of dropping to my heart only takes a second, and after a few more seconds in the heart, everything takes on a different perspective, but it does take consciousness and discipline to do it. It's much easier to explode! We have to be very aware of our immediate reaction, and once we notice it, use our will forces to say, "Stop! Drop to my heart and wait." And we need to breathe as we do it—a lot!

Try this next time you are about to snap back at someone; you might be surprised at how well things work out.

5. HAVE FAITH, TRUST AND COURAGE

If we held the faith that something full of love and wisdom and bigger than we can imagine is at work, that it has a plan spanning a far longer period than we can comprehend, how differently we would see our lives and respond.

What if we woke up every morning and said, "I will. I will to do Thy will," and then had the desire, courage, capacity and will to hold fast to that faith and trust? How different life would be if we could see the whole picture and not just our tiny little lives!

Have you ever reached a point where you exhausted yourself trying to fix everything for everyone and could do no more? Or you spent days caught in negative thoughts going round and round and finally gave up? And sure enough, when you let go and allowed God to step in and handle everything, it all worked out?

How many times have you limped through a life crisis, wondering why it is happening to you and feeling sorry for yourself, only to have insight several months or years later as to what was really going on?

Be courageous and know that we generally have no clue what is *really* going on! But if we tune in and pay attention, we may see glimpses of the phenomenal wisdom that is all around us, always. In the Bible, wisdom is called Sophia. Let her guide you. Have faith that that wisdom will work things out for the best. Listen for what you are guided to do, and do it!

WHAT WOULD KATHY DO?

Kathy finds a lot of things "interesting." Instead of an immediate panic reaction, she says to herself, "Interesting. I wonder what is really going on here. What is this really about? What is trying to emerge, arrive or unfold?"

My mentor Robert Sardello also has a wonderful way of reframing everything as interesting. Just that single approach can transform any situation, especially a potentially explosive one!

I have actually taught something similar for many years with this example: How many times has something happened or a phone call come in with bad news, and your immediate, visceral response has been, "Oh, no!" As soon as we shout out loud or silently "*Oh, no!*" a panic message is sent out to all our glands and we immediately release all sorts of stress chemicals that destroy any physiological calm we may have had.

But if we instead think to ourselves, "Oh, that's interesting" or "Okay, this is going to be an adventure!" a completely different reaction occurs in the body. There is no flood of adrenalin or cortisol, and we can calmly continue with curiosity! An added plus is that we keep breathing!

Kathy also uses the phrase, "Oh, well . . . it will all work out." That type of response also creates a very different state in our bodies—one of serenity as opposed to fear or panic about what may or may not happen.

It takes will *forces* (our part) and blessings (God's part) to behave in these ways, and will *power* and blessings to maintain a cheerful sense of certainty that things will actually work out. Many of the activities in this book are a new form of exercise for our will. We have different exercises for different muscle groups, and in the same way, we need different exercises to target specific aspects of our will not already developed.

To build will forces takes discipline. It takes commitment, effort and courage to hold onto faith, be in the heart, be cheerful, optimistic and hopeful at times of stress or difficulty, and be in a state of equanimity—but it's worth it!

With faith, trust, courage and blessings, take life as it comes, say, "Oh, that's interesting!" or "This is an adventure or mystery. I wonder what is really going on here. What is trying to emerge? What is the wisdom behind this? What is the big picture? What is my role?"

Or simply repeat, "It will all work out," instead of screaming in panic and running headlong into drama!

Easy!

6. LIVE IN HARMONY WITH THE RHYTHMS OF NATURE

When we feel well, care for ourselves and have reserves of love and energy from which we can draw to give to others, we are more joyful. If we lived life in harmony with the rhythms of nature that surrounded us—and we created rhythms in our own lives that grounded us, and returned us to our heart center—we would be developing the capacity of equanimity.

Rhythms or rituals can be something simple like having dinner together as a family; greeting each other with special kisses and hugs; taking walks in nature regularly; having weekly special baths; cleaning your face in a special way that nourishes you; reading inspirational material daily; or praying or meditating in a regular pattern.

The earth and every aspect of the human body are affected by the rhythms and cycles of the planets, cosmos, nature and seasons, to name only a few. Think of all the systems in nature that have rhythms and cycles—tides, sunrises, sunsets, the seasons, mating in animals, plants and their life cycles—everything in nature has a rhythm!

And we are part of that whole—our own body has cycles—women have menstrual cycles, men have hormonal cycles, we all have circadian rhythms that create optimal times of the day when our remedies or drugs will work more effectively amongst other things. I could go on for pages!

The point is that we are governed and surrounded by rhythms, and if we are in tune with them and create rituals to flow in harmony with nature's rhythms, we can be joyful, energized and composed, and life is easier.

Amen!

WHAT WOULD KATHY DO?

Kathy has her own inner state of rhythm. Tuned in and very sensitive to her surroundings, she is acutely aware of the importance of rhythms and rituals. She meditates daily and regularly makes time to do restorative and renewing activities.

Create your own routines and be conscious of nature's rhythms around you. Be active and dynamic and renew yourself in spring; enjoy the warmth of summer; shed the old in autumn; contract and build life forces in winter—only to blossom and bloom again in spring!

7. TAKE RESPONSIBILITY FOR YOUR OWN LIFE— LIVE WITH INTEGRITY

Imagine a world where we all took responsibility for our own actions and behaviors; a world where we accepted that we could only be responsible for our *own* lives, choices and decisions, and we allowed other adults the freedom to make their own choices, without judgment from us; a world where we loved others even if they made choices with which we did not agree.

All of this requires great maturity and equanimity and a much higher understanding of what really goes on in our world—knowing that what we actually perceive is just a tiny fraction of what there is to see.

So few people really take responsibility for themselves, their actions and their lives. They blame their parents, circumstances, teachers, siblings, the state, the government and even the weather. You name it, they blame it! Stop all blame now. Immediately! Blame, defensiveness and equanimity cannot coexist.

If you are blaming others or being defensive, look long and carefully at what you perceived them to do. Do you really think they intended to do what you think they did? Did they want to harm you? Did they know what they were doing? Did they on purpose destroy something for you? If they did, it's an opportunity for forgiveness! If not, it's a great chance for understanding and insight, which will change your perception.

And then look longer and more carefully at yourself! Did you do every-thing that you could possibly have done, with courage, integrity and honesty, to create a different scenario?

If you did the best you could, given your level of skills and knowledge, you can hold your head up high, so to speak, and there is no need for blame. You know you did your best, and you can, with composure, face what you need to face. If there was something more you could have done, learn from your mistakes and move on.

WHAT WOULD KATHY DO?

If you tell Kathy something in confidence, you know that no one—no one—will ever hear it from her. Not even her husband! Her integrity is impeccable.

How is your integrity?

Kathy is also a master at knowing what her responsibility is and taking action on it, and knowing clearly when responsibility lies with others. In that case, she lets them be responsible! And she stays in harmony, no matter what they do.

Gossip is not a responsible, compassionate, worthy or useful way to spend time. Do you take responsibility for what comes out of your mouth? No one else can be blamed for that! If you can walk around knowing that you have said nothing detrimental, harmful, unkind or negative, your path to equanimity will be faster.

Take some time to recognize patterns of blaming, defensiveness or reacting that have been created in your past. As you do this, you may be given different insights, which will allow you to change the patterns of behavior.

Do you do the "right" thing—even when no one is looking? Do you put grocery carts away even if they are not yours? Do you pick up clothes that fall to the floor in a store? Do you avoid parking in disabled car spaces? Do you always put money in parking meters? Do you keep your commitments?

I am pretty good at doing all those things—although I've been much better since I met my husband. (I never did park in handicapped spots, though!)

Our lives would be without guilt, defensiveness or fear of blame and accusations if we always did the right thing, if we lived with integrity in our hearts and if we were aware of the larger whole of which we are an integral part.

8. BE RECEPTIVE AND OPEN TO WHAT IS EMERGING

Most of us are generally unconscious of what is going on around us and within us—the spiritual currents, the nonverbal messages, the elements of nature, the influence of everything in the invisible soup in which we live. We are unaware of the grand plans of the spiritual wisdom that is operating.

It would seem wise to be open to the possibility that in every minute, spiritual elements are involved in forming us and shaping the world around us. If we can be interested and diligent observers and at the same time actively involved in what is going on and making our contribution, we are receptive and open.

When we are totally absorbed with ourselves, defending ourselves, judging, full of fear, living in the past, worrying about the future or disconnected from the whole, we cannot be receptive.

We need to be fully present in any situation in which we find ourselves. What does that mean?

It means we are in our hearts, fully conscious of the other person or people, the environment and the situation; free of any self-centered thoughts, worries or emotions about anything else; free of judgments, comparisons or idle chatter; and truly "with" whatever is going on.

Haven't you met people who listen to you in a way in which you really feel heard? You feel like they understand and care about you. You feel good around them. These are *present* people. Being present is being receptive.

When we are present (or receptive), we are open to what is there in the moment; we look with interest at *all* levels of communication and activity going on, at what might be unfolding and what might really be happening. We are interacting with others, but there is a part of us that is aware of the bigger picture and greater activity. Our perception is enhanced.

WHAT WOULD KATHY DO?

All of the above! Kathy has an incredible capacity for being present, patient, open, receptive and observant—at all levels. You would swear she is totally involved in every conversation, and she is—and at the same time, she is aware and conscious of everything else that is going on.

Kathy is so present that she can see when the other person is not. When she is saying something important that she really wants the other person to hear—and she has done this with me—she will hold their arms gently and look directly into their eyes. She then repeats herself, making sure that the listener really heard, absorbed and received the meaning and impact of the words she used! It is very powerful.

Of course, this has to be done with love and wisdom! We can't just grab someone and shout, "Listen to me—this is important!"

What we can do when we communicate is to make sure we look directly into the eyes of the person we are speaking with; be sure we have their attention and love in our heart, and then speak directly from our heart to theirs—via their eyes!

Kathy actively looks for what is emerging in a conversation—and that is key. You must have the intention of being receptive and open to anything that unfolds, actively seeking it, and have the courage to trust that you will be able to tap into your heart and deal with whatever happens.

It's also important to be discerning about what you are being receptive to, and act on your inspired intuition! A pure heart will only allow beneficial information in. It is very important to filter what we sense through a pure heart. If doubt arises, your heart is probably saying, "Check this out further!"

9. BE CONTENT AND CHOOSE YOUR FEELINGS

Have you ever been truly content and serene? I can only remember one moment in my life—I am sure there were more but I can only remember this one—of true contentment and absolute serenity, and I suspect, equanimity.

I was babysitting my adored Thomas and Clelia when they were about five and three. It was bath time, and while my nephew kept splashing, I had Clelia in my lap bundled up in a towel. I sat on the side of the bath, and a silence surrounded us. Clelia stopped squirming and my little nephew even stopped splashing, as time seemed to stop.

In that moment, every cell in my body knew—just *knew*—that everything was as it should be. All in the world was perfect, and I felt absolute peace and contentment. It was a fabulous experience. It lasted about twenty seconds. And soon we were back to splashing and laughing and running about—but I know we all felt it.

In my thinking, serenity and contentment go hand in hand. Are you content with your lot right now? If not, what is blocking your sense of being content? What can you do about it? If it's a person disrupting your peace, then are you allowing someone else to influence your emotions and state? Ultimately, only *you* can control how you react to your emotions!

Contrary to most psychological thinking and the children's song, "Sticks and stones will hurt my bones, but names can never hurt me," I believe people *can* emotionally hurt us. When people are emotionally or verbally abusive, cruel, alcoholic, manipulative or just moody, they *do* hurt our emotional body. Physical violence hurts both physical and emotional bodies. When anyone "hits" us in our emotional body, we can feel it.

To deal with the pain we have the capacity to forgive and move on, or do something about it. If we feel their intention was to make us angry or upset, we can check by asking, and say 'that made me angry or upset' and ask them to not do it again. If it was unintentional, we can communicate that it hurt and ask them to please be more careful in the future. Or we can pray for grace and the strength to forgive and move on. We are in control of whether we hang onto this hurt and pain in our emotional body and allow it to affect the rest of our lives—or not.

Remember—many events need not be emotionally stressful, but what we *tell ourselves* about them makes them either stressful or not. It's like the thunderstorm approaching the house. So who is in control of *your* emotions? Long-term, you!

You might think, "This situation is making me crazy," but really, it is *your reaction* that is driving you nuts! Take responsibility for your emotions and state of mind. Then take action to do something different: Remove yourself, change what you say to yourself about it, or go to your heart to seek help.

Examine why you are emotional and see if you can resolve what is causing it—and find the root of your discontent. It will probably be something *you* have been hanging onto, not something outside you!

10. CONTROL DESIRE AND COMPARISONS

One of the biggest enemies of equanimity is the tendency to compare ourselves with others. Materialism is rampant, and most people seem to want *more* of everything—more money, fame, power, control, possessions, clothes and so on. What happened to the simple life, when we were not consumed by material desires?

Isn't it interesting how the word "consumerism" is so common these days? In the simple life, we had only one television (GASP!), or we had only one phone, computer or car (or maybe two modest cars). Being overtaken by desires always leads to imbalance and misery and often to financial hardship.

We all yearn for connection to something greater than us. We may not realize this spiritual yearning, but deep inside our hearts, we yearn for that connection. It manifests as a sense of "There must be something more than this to life" or "Is this all there is?"

This yearning is often misinterpreted as a desire for something, so we try to accumulate as much as we can—money, power, fame, sex, stuff and relationships. Loneliness is at epidemic levels in the Western world and we know that loneliness and isolation cause disease: One recent poll reported that 4 in 10 Americans admit to frequent feelings of "intense loneliness."

In the simpler life, we recognized our desire was for a connection— with ourselves, our families and God. We spent more time with our families and connected more with them. We used to be more involved in our communities, and loneliness was not as common as it is now.

We had more communication face to face; our children did not stare at tiny little game screens, shooting and killing things while disconnecting completely from anyone around them. We were not addicted to computers and television. Our attention spans were longer than a gnat on speed!

Fewer people lived alone, and there were more multigenerational families. We grew our own food, cooked more meals and had fresh instead of processed foods every day. Meals were a connection time—not a series of staged microwaved meals eaten on the run.

We were, in short, physically and spiritually healthier and more content with our circumstances. We didn't always want more or bigger or better—all of which come from comparing what we have with what others have. Even if it is happiness or joy! And then we complain!

Stop comparing and complaining, and start making changes that will bring you joy: connect, pray, accept what you have, make the best of it and do the best you can. Do this and reconnect with God, yourself and others, and contentment and joy will be yours.

Or in closer reach anyway!

WHAT WOULD KATHY DO?

I don't know that I have ever heard Kathy complain. In all the time I have known her, she has never complained about anything. She might mention things with which she is dissatisfied, but in the same breath, she talks about what she is doing about it. Her life has not been especially easy and it is not perfect yet, but she is content with what she has and does.

She has worked very hard for a long time and is now making changes to allow a more relaxed lifestyle. She is active in creating her contentment. She makes the best of, and searches for the best in, every situation, no matter what it is.

I have never heard Kathy compare herself with anyone either!

I remember my precious mama telling me when I was small, "Comparisons are odious, darling!" Of course I had to ask her what that meant—but the phrase certainly stuck! And I was blessed to not have comparing as one of my personality traits.

Free yourself from comparisons, coveting and complaining, and find contentment and serenity!

This poem, "The Paradoxical Commandments," is from *Anyway* by Dr. Kent M. Keith. I thought it was a great way to finish a section on how to find equanimity.

People are illogical, unreasonable, and self-centered.
Love them anyway.
If you do good, people will accuse you of selfish ulterior motives.
Do good anyway.
If you are successful, you will win false friends and true enemies.
Succeed anyway.
The good you do today will be forgotten tomorrow.
Do good anyway.
Honesty and frankness make you vulnerable.
Be honest and frank anyway.
The biggest men and women with the biggest ideas can be shot down by
the smallest men and women with the smallest minds.
Think big anyway.
People favor underdogs but follow only top dogs.
Fight for a few underdogs anyway.
What you spend years building may be destroyed overnight.
Build anyway.
People really need help but may attack you if you do help them.
Help people anyway.
Give the world the best you have and you'll get kicked in the teeth.
Give the world the best you have anyway.[5]

DAILY SCHEDULE

SUNDAY: PEACE, PURE JOY AND HEARING GOD'S LAUGHTER

"Hafiz tells us that the Beloved's nature is pure joy, and the closer
we come to him, the more we are able to hear and feel God's
laughter. The rhythm of his laughter is the music of the dance
of life. That music is the essence of love and it is the radiant core
of every song of Hafiz. I am happy even before I have a reason."[6]

—Daniel Ladinsky

If God's nature is pure joy—so is yours! We are all made in His image,
so today is the day you feel joy "before you have a reason"! And let
laughter flow freely!

Pray before you climb out of bed, and ask God what He would like you to do this day! Then do it!

Be joyful just because you are by now, hopefully, more connected to God. Recognize the yearning or longing that has been in your heart for what it truly is—yearning for connection to God. Today—connect with Him. Look for moments to do that—through children, your family, strangers, nature or service.

Create, look for and find joyful moments all day. Make others smile, acknowledge them, accept them, laugh, let go and lighten up!

Skip, play, dance and sing for no reason. Ignore the judgments of others. Do stuff you love to do! Be kind, loving, gentle and helpful. Visit friends, hug someone, tell them you love them and be grateful for everything.

Go to bed thanking God on your knees for all that happened, and feel you did your best. If you could have done better, ask Him for another chance tomorrow.

Bathe in God's safety and love as you go to sleep!

MONDAY: FEEL COMPOSED AND PEACEFUL IN ALL SITUATIONS

"First, keep the peace within yourself, then you can also bring peace to others."

—Thomas À Kempis

Be conscious today of what you feel, what you are doing, and your motives. Are you taking responsibility for how you *feel*, what you do and what you say? Have you given responsibility for yourself or aspects of your life to others? Are you expecting others to make you feel better or good about yourself? You may be disappointed if that is the case!

Are you trying to manipulate a situation or others into doing things differently, or being different to suit your own needs and not theirs? Are you taking responsibility for another's life and conditions without being asked to help? Is it appropriate? Is this your job, really?

For a completely different perspective on why others are behaving as they are, think of a person you dislike intensely and put yourself in his or her shoes for today. If you do this sincerely, you may have a new way of understanding them and feel peaceful around them instead of wanting to kill them!

If you are not happy with your job, your relationship or any aspect of your life, take charge of your contribution to, and participation in, this situation, and what you say to yourself about it. Be very responsible with this exploration. Eliminate comparisons, be generous, be happy for others and share freely.

Are you happy with what you have? You might as well be, since it's what you have! You may desire more in your life or a change, but examine your desires: If they are all material—beware! If they all sound something like, "I want more money, a bigger house, a better car, more clothes, more power, more prestige, more things"—be very careful and explore a little deeper.

If your desires are centered around, "I want to serve and contribute more and be on purpose, following God's will or the divine plan for my life," then you are on track! And money will flow to you—the *more you give,* the more comes towards you. The more generous you are with your spirit and your possessions, the more contentment you will find.

If you find yourself rushing, worrying or stressed—stop, take a breath, drop to your heart, and stop the negative loop in your mind. Meditate, look at funny photos, or do something that you know will help you calm down. Also today be aware of negative emotions and any horses of emotion that are galloping around trying to carry you away. If you realize you are on a horse, immediately climb down and take charge of your emotional state!

Whatever mood you are in, you are in control of it. Choose to connect with God today and He will keep you composed and peaceful in every situation.

This could be a fun day! Your aim is to feel content the whole day.

TUESDAY: KNOW THE SPIRITUAL WORLD IS HERE, NOW, EVERYWHERE
Angels, fairies, elemental beings, tree spirits and animal spirits are everywhere. Invite them to speak to you today!

Your mission is to have faith and trust that everything in your life is touched and orchestrated to some degree by the divine. Examine from and with your heart all that is happening to you—all the dilemmas, difficulties, pain, good things and uncertainties—and see if you can find a bigger picture. Is there a reason this may be happening? Is there a lesson you need to be learning that you are currently not appreciating?

There is a higher wisdom and a bigger plan than you can comprehend. You may not understand, but you can still make sure you are doing what you are supposed to be doing to progress. If you cannot think of anything you are meant to be doing or learning, then ask God or your heart for guidance.

It takes an act of will and a lot of practice to go to your heart and stay there at all times. Most of us just wander around unconscious of the fact that we are being judgmental and out of balance. If we can stay in our hearts—or visit them as often as possible—we are in connection with the spiritual worlds—even if we don't know it!

Our hearts are our portals to the spiritual world. That's why the heart is so important for reconnecting with ourselves, God and others. Be patient, as it may take longer for the spiritual world to bring you what you need than you would like. Although sometimes it just happens suddenly!

So pray, be patient and look for the wisdom that is always there for you.

WEDNESDAY: BROTHERLY LOVE

Observe, don't judge; love instead. This is your mantra for today. If you find yourself judging someone, ask, "Am I perfect yet? Can I judge another?" and silently ask for that person's forgiveness and send them love. Know that you are them and they are you and we are all holograms of God.

Understand that every action you take and every word you say today will have an effect on everyone else around you, and probably on the planet as well. Consider that before you act and speak. Make every action and word loving.

Next time you are in a group, practice this by being present to the arguments, disagreements and differences, yet stay composed, accept the members as they are, and love them!

When you do throw something out the car window or toss litter on the street, you are separating yourself from the world. *Whatever* you do has an effect—even what you say to yourself! Make sure you have only a beneficial effect on everyone and everything today (and every day!).

Try to have some sense of that connection between you and all living things. Look at every plant and flower you pass today and thank it for giving you oxygen! Appreciate the rocks and any nature you may find around you.

It is a little harder in a concrete jungle of rushing, tense bodies but there are still moments you can find to feel connected, not with the tension and stress but with the deep silence, inner peace and love within every one of us—including ourselves.

Love your "brother." Everyone is your brother!

THURSDAY: RHYTHMS, RITUALS AND BEING RECEPTIVE

"Rhythm is the basis of life, not steady forward progress."

—The Kabbalah

Have a big day today! Step out this morning with the eyes of your heart open! Filter everything that happens to you through your heart and be receptive to what is unfolding in *every* situation. Be an involved observer. Catch yourself doing anything that would block receptivity and learning (judging, cynicism, fear, rushing, stress, worry), and drop to your heart to restore your receptivity.

If you notice doubt appearing, go immediately to your heart and ask questions. Explore your feelings further. Don't just shut down and judge. Have a sense that there are lessons for you in just about everything you are involved in, every day. Look for those lessons.

Be receptive to feelings of peace welling up from beneath your feet, being poured over your head and filling your heart! We are always showered with love and peace but don't know it. Today is the day to start receiving it and feeling it!

Make sure you are respectful of the rhythms of nature and your body. Sleep when it's dark, wake up early, and try to see more sunsets and sunrises—they are both filled with healing energies. Eat regularly, with consciousness and peace—not in the car, racing to work!

Take breaks when you're working. Find a rhythm between intense concentration and creative relaxation, and it will make your work much more effective. Try to find a park near work or a beautiful view or some place you can be and absorb the life forces nature and the sun gives you. Spend a little time every day in the sun if you can.

Create little rituals that help bring rhythm to your daily life. Have an unwind ritual on the way home so there is a separation between work and home. Have a dinner ritual. Meditate at the same time each day. Exercise each day.

I am sure you can think of many ways to restore some sense of rhythm that will also reconnect you to yourself and the rest of us!

FRIDAY: **FIND YOUR PURPOSE AND DO THE RIGHT THING**

"Make your work be in keeping with your purpose."

—Leonardo da Vinci

Are you fulfilling your purpose in life? Are you making a contribution of which you are proud? Do you have a nagging feeling that there is something you are meant to be doing and you're not? Are you feeling connected to yourself and God?

If you don't know what your life purpose is, make it a goal or your intention to find out. Pray about it, discuss it with your family, see vocational guidance people and search your heart—it will have the answers!

To help you identify your purpose, think of all the things you feel strongly about, care about a great deal or are passionate about. What makes you feel this way? Why are these things important to you? Are there other things to which you are indifferent, numb, resentful or passively aggressive? What has happened that you feel that way? If you don't care about certain things, ask yourself why. Think about why others would care about things you are not interested in.

Apart from pursuing your purpose with passion, what can you do to change the level of enthusiasm you feel? Be involved in your life—your work—your relationships—show up and participate enthusiastically. Do your part!

Be responsible, and if you are aware that you are allowing others to do what you are supposed to be doing, stop! Take charge of yourself! You are not a victim, and you need not be helpless or hopeless. You are an amazing spiritual being within a human body, and you need to live as that.

Let go of old stuff that is poisoning your spirit—release it and move on. No blame, no victim stuff—just stand up inside and have faith and courage, and start doing what you are supposed to be doing—or take steps in that direction. Begin your journey in some way today.

Do the right thing today—be of the highest character, be trustworthy and honorable, and act with integrity, even if no one else is watching or will know about it.

YOU will know.

SATURDAY: BE YOUR TRUE SELF AND TRULY KNOW OTHERS

We are all like a single cell in a body—intricately connected to, and affecting, everything else. It's important to understand what sort of cell you are, do your job and act in harmony with every other cell—whether close to you or trillions of cells away. Imagine the impact you have on all of them and the impact every other cell has on you.

Spend this day suspending all opinions, judgments and ideas about other people—and yourself! Try to tap into the *real* you—the one in your heart that God sees, uncolored by upbringing, parents, siblings and life to date. Dwell on (or find out) what is important to you, what you really value, what or who really excites you and stirs your passion, and what or who drains you, and see any patterns of behavior that you feel really aren't the real you. Is there a "trapped" you inside waiting to emerge?

Write, "Who am I?" at the top of a page, and then describe who you think you are—not what you do but who you *are*. Ask your partner to do this as well!

With others, try to see them today as *they* really are. Look with your true heart and see the person who is your wife, husband or partner—check to see if you are really seeing an ex-partner as you look at them or are projecting other qualities onto them and treating them as if they were someone else. Think very carefully on this one—*feel* into it. It is often difficult to be aware that you are doing this.

How well do you know your partner? Both of you can write a list of, "Who do I think my partner is?" and then compare notes! Do you really know what is important to them? Do you really understand them? With time (and possibly some counseling!), you may discover a whole new person!

Maybe this project will take a little longer than a day! LOL.

But today is a great start!

EPILOGUE

Everything always depends on the way in which things are done—what we do, how we do it and *the spirit in which we do it*.

The *activity* and the *results* are also important! We must pray to do it right, take action in the right spirit, and God will provide the resources and make a great outcome possible. Our job is to use our gifts and talents to *serve* and *help* others where we can. We are always planting seeds. It's about having the *right* spirit, asking for the *right* blessings and then *doing* the *right* thing!

"Do unto others as you would have them do unto you."

—Luke 6:31

Do the things in this book, and the spirit of joy will fill your life.

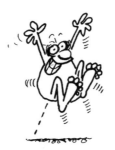

SUMMARY OF THE EXERCISES FOR EACH WEEK

Chapter 1: **GRATITUDE**
SUNDAY: Gratitude to God
MONDAY: Workplace gratitude
TUESDAY: Home gratitude
WEDNESDAY: "The past" gratitude
THURSDAY: Body gratitude
FRIDAY: Nature gratitude
SATURDAY: Heart gratitude

Chapter 2: **COMPASSION/GRACE**
SUNDAY & MONDAY: Self-less-ness
TUESDAY: Compassion for your boss, colleagues and customers
WEDNESDAY & THURSDAY: Compassion at home
FRIDAY: Compassion for your "enemies"
SATURDAY: Compassion for yourself

Chapter 3: **HOPE**
SUNDAY: Hope and faith
MONDAY: Find where hope lives in your body
TUESDAY: Hope for yourself
WEDNESDAY: Find the fears, move to hope
THURSDAY: Hopeful expectations
FRIDAY: Tackle something difficult with hope
SATURDAY: The difference between hope-ing and hope-ful

Chapter 4: **REVERENCE**

SUNDAY: Reverence for God, our angels and all the spiritual beings who help us
MONDAY: Reverence for life
TUESDAY: Reverence for nature
WEDNESDAY: Reverence for others
THURSDAY: Reverence for your soul and spirit
FRIDAY: Reverence for your body
SATURDAY: Reverence for your food

Chapter 5: **GENEROSITY, GIVING AND RECEIVING**

SUNDAY: Be generous with your spirit
MONDAY: Be generous with your time
TUESDAY: Give from your heart
WEDNESDAY: Give to yourself and receive it
THURSDAY: Give your blessings
FRIDAY: Receive, with grace
SATURDAY: Ask and receive

Chapter 6: **FORGIVENESS**

SUNDAY: Forgive them for they know not what they do
MONDAY: Breaking the bonds
TUESDAY: Ask for forgiveness
WEDNESDAY: Let go of embarrassment and shame
THURSDAY: Forgive yourself
FRIDAY: The other person's response
SATURDAY: Apologize

Chapter 7: **ENERGY AND VITALITY**

SUNDAY: Spiritually reenergize
MONDAY: Eating and drinking patterns and routines
TUESDAY: Be conscious of what you drink
WEDNESDAY: Be conscious of how much you move
THURSDAY: Sleep and energy

FRIDAY: Bust stress
SATURDAY: Energy givers and suckers

Chapter 8: **LISTENING**
SUNDAY: Listen to God
MONDAY: Listen with your heart for feelings and let people feel safe with you
TUESDAY: Why am I battering myself?
WEDNESDAY: Listen to your heart
THURSDAY: Listen with discernment and speak only good
FRIDAY: Ask questions
SATURDAY: Disguises that words take on

Chapter 9: **LAUGHTER**
SUNDAY: Smile and stop taking yourself so seriously
MONDAY: Remember all the funny times in your life
TUESDAY: Find photos of as many fun times as you can
WEDNESDAY: Watch a movie that makes you laugh out loud
THURSDAY: Laugh and help others laugh
FRIDAY: Make a laughter journal and read funny stuff
SATURDAY: Turn around tough memories with laughter

Chapter 10: **LOVE**
SUNDAY: Love God
MONDAY: Be a love ray-diator! Think only loving thoughts
TUESDAY: Loving actions
WEDNESDAY: Love your life
THURSDAY: Give everyone TA-DA's
FRIDAY: Love yourself
SATURDAY: Hold people in your heart

Chapter 11: **CHEERFUL ENTHUSIASM**
SUNDAY: Look for miracles
MONDAY: Choose your moods

TUESDAY: Face all your difficulties with cheerfulness
WEDNESDAY: Be passionate about being enthusiastic
THURSDAY: Smile all day—at everyone!
FRIDAY: Always think with a joyful heart that things will steadily improve
SATURDAY: Find your work

Chapter 12: **EQUANIMITY**
SUNDAY: Peace, pure joy and hearing God's laughter
MONDAY: Feel composed and peaceful in all situations
TUESDAY: Know the spiritual world is here, now, everywhere
WEDNESDAY: Brotherly love
THURSDAY: Rhythms, rituals and being receptive
FRIDAY: Find your purpose and do the right thing
SATURDAY: Be your true self and truly know others

RESOURCES

AMANDA GORE: To book for speaking engagements and for all other inquiries, email amanda@amandagore.com.

Endorphins, magic wands, gratitude glasses, joy journals, books and zoots are available on our website: www.amandagore.com.

LYME TESTING: www.centralfloridaresearch.com/lab
LYME RESEARCH: www.samento.com, www.neuraltherapy.com
SCHOOL OF SPIRITUAL PSYCHOLOGY: www.spiritualschool.org
Wonderful classes and books. Co-founded by Robert and Cheryl Sardello.
MICHAEL GRINDER: www.michaelgrinder.com
Excellent books, programs and classes on group dynamics, nonverbal communication and leadership.
LARRY BYRAM: www.higheralignment.com
Excellent information about communication and relationship styles, and many other aspects of joy.
JOHN GOTTMAN: www.gottman.com
Emeritus professor of psychology at the University of Washington and co-founder of The Gottman Institute.
HEARTMATH: www.heartmath.com
Interesting research on the heart; stress management programs; enhanced performance. www.heartmath.com
BYRON KATIE: www.thework.com

RECOMMENDED BOOKS

Silence Robert Sardello
The Power of Soul Robert Sardello
Freeing the Soul from Fear Robert Sardello
Love and the Soul Robert Sardello
I Heard God Laughing: Poems of Hope and Joy Daniel Ladinsky
The Gift: Poems by Hafiz Daniel Ladinsky
The People Pill Ken Wright
Dangerous Grains James Braly and Ron Hoggan
Healing Lyme Stephen Harrod Buhner
Celiac Disease: A Hidden Epidemic Peter Green and Rory Jones
Man's Search for Meaning Viktor Frankl
Turning Claire Blatchford
Becoming Claire Blatchford
Friend of My Heart Claire Blatchford
Illusions Richard Bach
The Bridge Over the River Translated by Joseph Wetzl
The Seven Principles for Making Marriage Work
     John Gottman and Nan Silver
Sweet Deception Dr. Joseph Mercola
Aspartame Disease: An Ignored Epidemic H.J. Roberts
Molecules of Emotion Candace Pert
The Seven Habits of Highly Effective People Stephen R. Covey
Nourishing Traditions Sally Fallon
The Heart's Code Paul Pearsall
Dave Barry Turns 40 Dave Barry

NOTES

FRONT MATTER

1. From *The Bridge Over the River: After-Death Communications of a Young Artist Who Died in World War I*; (Sigwart Botho Phillip August Eulenburg), translated by Joseph Wetzl; Anthroposophic Press, N.Y.)

CHAPTER 1

1. From *Friend of My Heart: Meeting Christ in Everyday Life* by Claire Blatchford (1999) Lindisfare: Hudson, N.Y.

2. From *Worldly Virtues: A Catalogue of Reflections* by J. A. Gaertner (2002). Excerpted with permission of Phanes Press, imprint of Red Wheel/Weiser; www.redwheel weiser.com. To order, call 800.423.7087.

3. Susan L. Taylor, editor of *Essence* magazine and author of *In the Spirit: The Inspirational Writings of Susan L. Taylor.*

4. Rabbi Harold Kushner, author of *When Bad Things Happen to Good People* and *How Good Do We Have to Be?*

5. Helen Keller, author of *The Light in My Darkness,* published by Chrysalis: West Chester, Penn.

6. Playwright Bertolt Brecht, from the play *Jungle of Cities,* 1924.

CHAPTER 2

1. From *The Dalai Lama: My Tibet* by the Dalai Lama; the University of California Press, (1990). Used by permission.

2. From *The Asian Journal of Thomas Merton* by Thomas Merton (1975), New York: New Directions.

3. From *The Wisdom Teachings of the Dalai Lama* by Matthew E. Bunson (1997); Used by permission of Dutton, a division of Penguin Group (USA) Inc.

CHAPTER 3

1. From *A Long Obedience in the Same Direction: Discipleship in an Instant Society* by Eugene H. Peterson. (1998) Downers Grove, IL: InterVarsity Press. Reprinted with permission.

CHAPTER 4

1. From *I Heard God Laughing: Poems of Hope and Joy* by Daniel Ladinsky; Penguin. "My Brilliant Image" by Hafiz, translated by Daniel Ladinsky (1996; 2006) Reprinted with permission.

2. Don Coyhis of the Mohican Nation; president and co-founder of White Bison Inc.; www.whitebison.org; 719.548.1000. Reprinted with permission.

3. From *I Heard God Laughing: Poems of Hope and Joy*, Hafiz, translated by Daniel Ladinsky; 1996; 2006, Penguin. Reprinted with permission.

CHAPTER 6

1. From "Some Notes on Forgiveness as an Act of Love" by Robert Sardello; School of Spiritual Psychology E-letter," (Jan. 2002); www.spiritualschool.org

CHAPTER 7

1. From *The Future of Love* by Daphne Rose Kingma; (1999). Berkeley; Main Street Books. Reprinted with permission.

2. Eve Van Cauter, Professor of Medicine, University of Chicago. Reprinted with permission of the Department of Medicine, University of Chicago.

3. Dr. Sanjay R. Patel of Harvard Medical School. Quoted in an article by Rob Stein, *Washington Post,* October 9, 2005.

CHAPTER 8

1. From *Practicing the Sacred Art of Listening* by Kay Lindahl; (www.sacredlistening.com) Reprinted with permission.

2. From *I Heard God Laughing: Poems of Hope and Joy* by Daniel Ladinsky; 1996; 2006, Penguin. Reprinted with permission.

3. U.S. State Department spokesman Robert McCloskey during one of his regular noon briefings during the worst days of the Vietnam War, quoted by Marvin Kalb in *TV Guide,* March 31, 1984.

CHAPTER 9

1. From *I Heard God Laughing: Poems of Hope and Joy,* Hafiz, translated by Daniel Ladinsky; 1996; 2006, Penguin. Reprinted with permission.

CHAPTER 10

1. From *Becoming: A Call to Love* by Claire Blatchford; (2004) Lindisfarne; Hudson, N.Y.

2. From *364 Days of Love* by Daphne Rose Kingma, (1992); Conari Press, Berkeley, CA: Reprinted with permission.

CHAPTER 11

1. *The Bridge Over the River,* Vol. 2, from an unpublished manuscript translated by Joseph Wetzl. All effort was made to find the author and seek permission. We apologize if there is any infringement. Please contact us. www.amandagore.com.

2. Ibid.

CHAPTER 12

1. Excerpt from the Penguin anthology, *Love Poems from God,* by Daniel Ladinsky (2002). Reprinted with permission.

2. From an unpublished lecture in Bremen, Germany on Dec. 12, 1911, by Rudolf Steiner: "Death and Immortality in the Light of Spiritual Science."

3. From *Powers Within: Selections from the Works of Sri Arubindo and the Mother;* compiled by A. S. Dalal; published by Lotus Press.

4. John 4:12 No one has seen God at any time; if we love one another, God abides in us, and His love is perfected in us. 4:13 By this we know that we abide in Him and He in us, because He has given us His spirit.

John 3:14-17 We know that we have passes out of death into life, because we love the brethern. He who does not love abides in death. Everyone who hates is brother is a murderer; and you know that no murderer has eternal life abiding in him. We know love by this, that He laid down His life for us; and we ought to lay down our lives for the brethern. But whoever has the world's goods, and sees his brother in need and closes his heart against him, how does the love of God abide in him?

5. *Anyway: The Paradoxical Commandments—Finding Personal Meaning in a Crazy World* by Dr. Kent M. Keith and Spencer Johnson; (1968, 2001); Reprinted with permission.

6. From *I Heard God Laughing: Poems of Hope and Joy* by Daniel Ladinsky; 1996; 2006, Penguin. Reprinted with permission.

WHO IS AMANDA GORE?

Amanda Gore is a blessed person!

For 25 years Amanda has been inspiring groups worldwide with humor, honesty and her simple, effective lessons, some of which you can read about in this book. Amanda's background in physical therapy, psychology, neurolinguistics, ergonomics and group dynamics has created a unique platform for her motivational speaking career.

For more information, to purchase other books or products or to book Amanda to speak at your conference, visit www.amandagore.com.

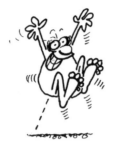